The Complete Guide
to a
Dynamic Body

by Karen Lustgarten

photography by
BERNIE LUSTGARTEN

FAWCETT COLUMBINE • NEW YORK

Other Books by the Same Author:

The Complete Guide to Disco Dancing

The Complete Guide to Touch Dancing

THE COMPLETE GUIDE TO A DYNAMIC BODY

Published by Fawcett Columbine Books, a unit of CBS
Publications, the Consumer Publishing Division of CBS Inc.

ISBN: 0-449-90016-9

Printed in the United States of America

First Fawcett Columbine printing: May 1980

10   9   8   7   6   5   4   3   2   1

DEDICATION

To Bernie Lustgarten

for giving his constant friendship

and part of his soul to this work,

and

to Ruth Miller for believing in it.

ACKNOWLEDGMENTS

Over six years have passed since Bernie Lustgarten and I set out to work on this book. My dream of our collaborating to make this an exceptional, aesthetic work could not have come to fruition if it weren't for Bernie's photography talent, his intelligence, and his understanding patience with my unconventional ideas. Despite the passing of time, a divorce, and the publication of two other books on dance, this work retains sentimental feelings. It represents my very first collaboration with Bernie and the beginning of our mutual admiration and lifelong friendship.

Over five years ago Ruth Miller, editor at the *San Francisco Chronicle,* gave me my first break by accepting these exerises as a weekly newspaper column. Due to her efforts, the column has been running continuously ever since, and even enjoyed syndication for a time under her glorious title, "The Dynamic Body." Her enthusiasm for my exercise technique convinced many friends and co-workers at the *Chronicle* to enroll in my classes. I'm deeply indebted to Ruth for her belief in my work and constant support of it; but ultimately I'm grateful for the precious friendship of such a wonderful colleague.

Whether "sexy exercise" partner in this book or dancing partner in my other books, Ivan Ladizinsky is the bionic man who has succeeded in making his body grow younger. At age forty-six(!), Ivan is a busy executive who serves as an inspiration to anyone believing that fitness over forty is a fantasy. I thank him for being my personal inspiration and special person.

Finally, I'm truly indebted to my exercise students, especially those in the advanced class, who have been requesting over the years that I write this book. Observing their improvement from beginner to advanced level and experiencing their enthusiasm and appreciation for my Technique have been great sources of personal satisfaction and encouragement!

CONTENTS

PREFACE

Watch leaves reach, twist, undulate, and sway gracefully in courtship with the breeze. The limbs are supportive, strong, and dependable in the face of mood changes. Feel skipping water twirl, flow, and splash with delicate grace. It uncurls and stretches out for the sand. Birds glide freely and joyously suspended in weightless buoyancy. Everywhere we are surrounded by nature's beauty, strength, and grace, balanced and coordinated in its art works.

Nowhere is nature's beauty harmonized and so dramatically appreciated as it is in the human body. At their peak, our bodies possess the same harmony, grace, and strength that flow through the rest of nature. The exquisite science of the human body is in the static form that it takes. The poetry is in its dynamic movements. To a great extent, *we* are the sculptors of our own living forms.

The method that we all use in creating a work of art from our bodies is called body conditioning, or exercise—a method of improving the condition of our muscles and tendons so that our bodies take on aesthetic lines and shapes. A conditioned body takes on the form of a sculptured silhouette: firm, taut, toned, trimmed, strong, and pliant. A conditioned body also exudes a dynamic ability. It moves with spontaneous grace, with unrestricted freedom, with elegant carriage. It breathes vitality and agility in its flow with nature. It is light, graceful, and coordinated.

In addition to form and function, body conditioning effects a change in personality. We feel a joy and gratification in free, loose, boundless motion. We are energized and animated in daily living. As the body blooms in health, we open and flower in our personal relationships. We develop a new purpose and pride in using muscles. The art of body conditioning permeates all aspects of our lives—our physical form, the quality of our movement, and our feelings of well-being. We feel *deeply* alive.

To express my philosophy that the body is really nature's work of art, I have attempted to produce a truly beautiful exercise book. All of the exercises were photographed by Bernie Lustgarten with aesthetics, variety, and joy in mind. We spent nearly four years photographing outdoors and indoors, hoping to capture the artistic beauty of an active human body so that our readers would feel inspired to take action. The use of line drawings, vapid or clinical settings, and unimaginative exercises was automatically rejected for this book. Instead, Bernie and I set out to explore Northern California for backgrounds that would harmonize with each exercise. We found naturally twisted trees that emulated the shape and pose of an exercise; and we located wall graphics, sand dunes, sculptures, and playgrounds that provided complementary backgrounds for a particular body pose. In keeping with our "natural" philosophy, none of the photographs have been retouched.

In addition to visual interest, I wanted to create an intelligent, purposeful, and enjoyable exercise technique that would appeal to all levels of ability, from beginner through advanced, without danger of injury at any level. Most people aren't aware that exercises can be harmful to one's health unless they are performed correctly and we know the benefits and goals of each one. Therefore, I created a "Body Awareness" section for each exercise to help you understand and practice the correct way to use your muscles.

Throughout my athletic and dance years, I have never considered exercise to be a boring drudgery. On the contrary, I've found it to be a joyous expression and release of my physical, mental, and emotional self. Besides, all that effort has had bonus rewards: creating a refined living sculpture out of one's own body.

I am writing this book for everyone who has searched for the key to one of nature's most beautiful treasures—possession of a dynamic, glowing, conditioned body every joyous day of our lives. The treasure is buried within each of us.

HOW TO BEGIN ETC

The quickest, most reliable way to attain a conditioned and dynamic body is by conscious, intelligent exercising of your muscles. Body conditioning is both a science and an art. It requires your patience (the process cannot be hurried), consistency, time, and determined effort in the form of physical exertion. Each chapter in this book deals with a different part of the body so that you can select the exercises that fit your own personal conditioning needs and target any specific area. In reality, our muscles and body sections function interdependently: one stomach exercise may also be working muscles of the back, waist, thighs, etc. For this reason I have described, in the case of every exercise, those other body parts that are involved in performing any exercise.

Quality vs. Quantity

If your goal is a total, well-conditioned body, you'll need to use every muscle correctly. I emphasize correctness here because the *quality* of your movements (how you move) is even more important than the quantity (how much) or the speed (how fast) you move. Unless an exercise is performed knowledgeably, with attention to body alignment and placement, you'll be wasting your time creating strains and tensions where they shouldn't be. Even worse, you could be creating defects. For example, if you attempt a stomach exercise by allowing the muscles to protrude, then you'll be training your stomach to protrude! You won't be just "bending down," but bending in a specified way so you can extract maximum benefit for the muscles involved. To give another example, one common exercise to stretch the back and hamstring muscles is this forward bend. Performed correctly, this exercise is an extremely beneficial stretch, and it can also tone the stomach and waistline. Performed incorrectly, it will give you a rounded back, a pain in the neck (and shoulders) and hyperextended knees.

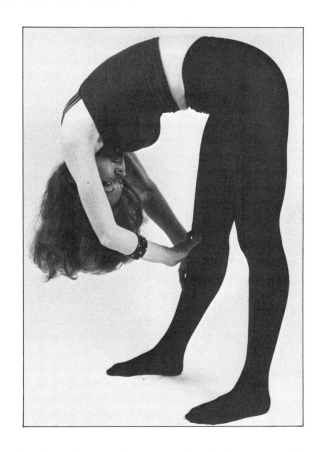

In the above photo my back is rounded, my shoulders are bunched up to my ears (causing the neck to tense), my stomach is lax and my weight is more toward my heels (putting too much pressure on my knees). I'm doing more harm than good by training my shoulders and back to round. Yet most people exercise this way!

To correct the position, pull the stomach in, straighten the back, keep the shoulders down and relaxed, and place your weight more toward the front part of the feet (see photo). Now you're correctly training the back to straighten and you're receiving the full stretch benefit for your muscles.

So important is this awareness and sensing of the correct way to align and move your body, that I have guided you throughout every exercise in three places.

First, under the "Position" heading, you're aligning your body parts in preparation for the exercise.

If the muscles are going to perform accurately and smoothly, they'll need to be in correct alignment before you even begin.

Next, the actual description of performing the exercise emphasizes how to best condition the target area at each level of ability (beginners, intermediates, and advanced).

Then, in the "Body Awareness" section, special attention is given to help you develop a kinesthetic awareness of the correct position, control, and coordination of other muscles when they orchestrate. Only by consciously sensing and placing the dynamic body parts where they should be can you derive any real benefit from any exercise.

Finally, each chapter ends with a section of "secret exercises." Just as there is a right way of performing an exercise, so there is a certain alignment when we move about during our daily activities that will tone and condition our bodies. The way we stand, sit, or walk through life contributes to or detracts from the condition of our muscles. This section offers guidance in consciously training our bodies to (habitually) apply all the conditioning techniques to routine living (without looking like we're actually exercising) so that we can enjoy a more dynamic body.

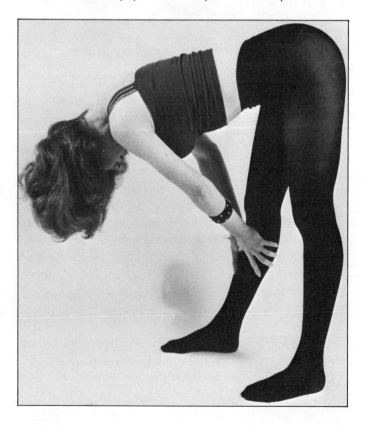

Meet Your Muscles

Once you've been exercising regularly, you may notice a slight weight gain even though you've lost inches. Muscle tissue weighs more than fatty tissue, but takes up less room. An inactive muscle will lose its firmness, turn to flab, and spread. To replace this fatty tissue with muscle tissue, you'll need to exercise. The only way you can make your body firm and compact is to reduce fatty tissue by increasing muscle tissue. Exercise will make the muscle grow in size (become heavier) and take up the loose slack, creating a defined curve where there was once a hanging sack.

We own about 639 muscles, composed of fibers that need to receive nerve impulses to tell them how to move. We make our moves whenever muscles shorten (contract), extend, become elastic (stretch and return), and grow (increase in width). At their fullest potential they are flexible and strong. A toned muscle needs 40 percent less energy to accomplish the same task as weak, flabby muscle. So whenever you tire from simple tasks or short exercise periods, it's because your muscles aren't in top condition.

Muscles will adapt to the amount of work (stretching and strengthening) demanded from them, but your demands must be increased gradually and consistently. As they adapt to one level, your efforts can be increased. If you overload them with too much work, the fibers will pull apart or tear, and you'll be at the mercy of time and rest until they mend. Muscles are basically a recalcitrant medium, but they will respond to your efforts. The appropriate exercises, done gradually, consistently, and correctly, will produce the rewards of physical refinement you seek.

Before you plunge into conditioning your muscles, there are some guidelines and cautions. If you're over 35 or have never been physically active, or have become active only recently, be sure to consult a doctor before selecting exercises. The same applies to anyone who is obese or under severe emotional stress.

Assuming that you have your doctor's clearance, you'll want to begin by evaluating your own conditioning needs, then setting realistic goals based on your present level of ability. Ability depends on heredity, mental attitude, and the extent and kind of previous exercise. All the exercises in these chapters are written so that you can progress to a higher level of ability. My advice is always to start with the beginner level and build slowly from there. Don't be overanxious for quick results. Be satisfied with gradual, steady improvements. If you make exercise a daily habit, then gradual consistency will bring you physical joys. Sporadic attempts will always fail.

There's no reason to consider exercise a drudgery, especially if you follow some of the suggestions below. Most important is to *enjoy* the delicious sensation of using your muscles every day, and of looking and feeling animated.

Begin by carving out a section of time *each* day just to exercise. This is your exclusive, uninterrupted, private time for tuning in to your physical self. Face it, the body's need for activity cannot be postponed to weekends only. So pick a time of day when you'll have privacy for ten minutes (beginners) and increase the time gradually to 20 minutes and eventually to 60 minutes as stamina and ability and interest improve. Stop when boredom or fatigue start to appear. Try to avoid times following a meal (allow at least 1½–2 hours after eating), or immediately upon waking when muscles are their stiffest.

Look and feel attractive for your exercise session. Some people enjoy preceding their session with a hot bath or shower to relax the muscles first. Now carve a special space for yourself in a warm room (no drafts, but not stuffy either). You might like to go all the way and make the room fragrant with flowers, perfume, or incense. Wear little or no clothes (leotard and tights or shorts), so you can watch your muscles. If possible, try to exercise in front of a full-length mirror so you can correct your placement and alignment and see and feel each movement. One way to avoid monotony is by choosing a variety of exercises. I've given you 125 exercises, each with its own feeling, form, and purpose. Plan to spend at least 2 minutes on each one, and work up to 3 minutes each. Also, try playing your favorite rhythmic music, and let your movement punctuate the rhythm. Occasionally, try exercising with a friend (see Chapter Seven: Sexy Exercises).

Expect to feel some temporary muscle soreness in the form of stiffness, especially if you haven't used certain muscles in years, or if you're working at a more advanced level. Soreness can be minimized by taking a hot bath or shower immediately preceding or following a session. Then slowly, gently, rhythmically repeat the same exercise each day that instigated soreness.

If you begin each session with warm-up stretches for at least 5 minutes, then you can reduce soreness and prepare your muscles for activity to follow (see: Roof Reach, Pinwheels, Windmill Lunge, Warm-up Bounces, Jumping Rope,). The idea is to raise your heartbeat and the temperature of your muscles, since warm muscles are 20 percent more efficient, and more elastic, therefore less vulnerable to aches and pulls. Add a few strengtheners for toning, some vigorous overall conditioners, and end with a few relaxers.

Work up to your own limit of stretch and strength, but don't overstrain, and please don't hold your breath! If you feel a cramp (a sudden muscle contraction or spasm where the muscle isn't relaxed or conditioned), then stop and gently pound on it with both fists, or knead the area with both hands, to increase the circulation to the area. If you happen to skip three weeks or more of exercising, then go back to the beginning, and don't expect to return to your previous level of ability for at least three weeks!

While you're exercising, make your movements smooth, fluid, and fresh, never stiff, jerky, or mechanical. To keep a rhythmic flow, I strongly suggest exercising to music of your preference. Any work or exercise is easier to do, and is done more efficiently, when it is performed to a distinct rhythm. Keep the music playing as you move in a continuous smooth flow without pausing too long between sets or exercises. At first you should build a routine (see Chapter Nine: The Lustgarten Technique). Later, seek variety in exercises as you increase your stamina, flexibility, and strength.

Your progress will depend on the intensity and duration of your efforts and on the quality of your movements. Just because a workout is strenuous won't guarantee that it's an effective one, especially if it is done in a perfunctory or half-hearted manner without attention to posture (body alignment) and the exercise goal. Try not to concentrate on the number of your repetitions. In fact, don't even bother counting at all. Instead, perform an exercise until you feel that you've reached your limit of ability, and concentrate on your alignment and the quality of your movements.

Rewards and Benefits

Besides the visible physical rewards, exercise will produce some unexpected psychological benefits. We know that it eases mental and emotional stress. It gives us an invigorating lift by releasing nervous tension, acting as a natural tranquilizer. It dispels sedentary fatigue, the kind that overcomes us when we are bored or when our torpid muscles crave rejuvenation after a physically inactive day at the office, at home, or at school.

We know that regular exercise can reduce symptoms relating to hypokinetic diseases (caused by insufficient motion): back pain, nervous tension, heart trouble, obesity, emotional stress, headaches, even colds and sore throats. Finally, exercise has other physiological benefits in that it improves the tissues and the functioning of the organs. Since it makes the heart more efficient, the risk of heart attacks is diminished. Blood pressure, heart rate, and cholesterol levels are all lowered. So is our weight and the amount of fat stored. Even the aging process can slow down.

Exercise can also increase sexual enjoyment and ability. It can heighten our awareness of ourselves and our own presence. It makes us respond with greater alertness. Without exercise, our muscles shrink in size, lose strength, become stiff. The heart shrinks in size, becomes weaker, and is less efficient. Eventually the symptoms of hypokinetic diseases creep into our bodies.

If you want the very most from life, then you will simply set aside time for exercising, just as you do for eating, sleeping, and working. Eventually you'll begin to feel that a day without exercise is an incomplete day. We need not live a sedentary life of sloth and physical deterioration due to inactivity. We really *can* rejuvenate our fossilized, crystallized bodies to salubrious heights by feeling the joy of our own strength, flexibility, and ease of movement. As we awaken our muscles from their sleep and discover the amazing abilities that lie within our own body, we can grow deeply alive. Let's begin!

CHAPTER ONE:

HOW TO SHRINK YOUR STOMACH AND WAIST

A firm, fabulous waistline—two wedge-shaped indentations in the male, or two long, graceful concave curves in the female—is associated with a youthful, active body. A thin waistline is usually accompanied by a flat stomach, sometimes defined so clearly as to take on a "washboard" effect. But a firm middle accented on either side by two smooth, narrow indentations is not associated so much with youth as it is with activity. When the midriff muscles lose their tone due to inactivity, the upper torso turns from trim triangle to thick rectangle. That "washboard" of muscular definition gives way to a cascading ripple of bulges and rolls in the middle, and spreads into a spare tire.

If I had to choose only one section of my entire body to condition daily, it would be my stomach. Your stomach really holds the key to your posture and balance, and it provides support to the entire upper body, helping to keep your back straight. Although the abdomen extends from the chest to the groin, the weakest muscles are usually in your lower abdomen—that area between your navel and groin. Good old gravity is constantly coaxing downward all the organs that lie behind your abdominal wall: the intestines, colon, liver, and stomach. If the upper and lower abdominal muscles are weak, gravity wins the constant tug of war, and your abdominal contents start spilling downward, forming a forward bulge smack-dab in your middle. If the upper and lower abdominal wall is kept strong and flat, the contents can be kept well contained and positioned within it.

If you seriously want to shrink the rolls around your waist and abdominal area, besides dieting you'll need to constantly strengthen your abdominals and stretch your waistline. One of the most effective ways to accomplish this is to draw in your stomach for the rest of your life! Stand in front of a mirror and pull in your stomach, then lift it up a bit. Notice how your waistline narrows and your abdomen flattens? Now relax your shoulders and retract your stomach only to the point where you can still breathe normally. Although this may not be the most comfortable way to go about life, it is the very best stomach exercise you can do to keep your midriff muscles in condition. Honestly, what benefit can you derive from huffing and puffing through 100 sit-ups

if the rest of your waking hours are spent just letting it all hang out?

Although any of the stomach strengtheners serve as good waist-shaping exercises, you can also trim your waist by stretching the side and lower-back muscles, and with reaching, twisting, and sidestretching exercising. Consistent sidestretching and twisting can quickly shave down a pair of "handlebars," and a little toning goes a long way in deflating a spare tire and central swell.

All of the exercises in this chapter target your waist and addominal muscles, which will quickly deteriorate from disuse. However, in most other exercises in this book, you'll notice that I have you draw your stomach in while you're exercising, making *every* exercise an abdominal toner! By hook or by crook, my program will help shrink your stomach and waist!

The Technique: Stomach Strengtheners

Leg-downs

Stomach "do's and don'ts":
One common method for strengthening the stomach muscles is with "leg-ups," in which both legs are raised from the floor simultaneously. Unfortunately, most instruction does not specify *how* to raise your legs so that you derive stomach benefits. If your stomach muscles are somewhat weak already, you won't be able to lift both legs without arching your lower back off the floor. Now you're really using your lower back to perform the exercise, and you're putting too much of a strain on the lower-back vertebrae. By arching, you're also allowing your stomach to pop out. Instead of training your stomach muscles to flatten, you're actually training them to protrude while you're inviting low-back pain! The correct way to perform the exercise is to melt your lower back to the floor, flatten your stomach, then hold the position while you lift your legs.

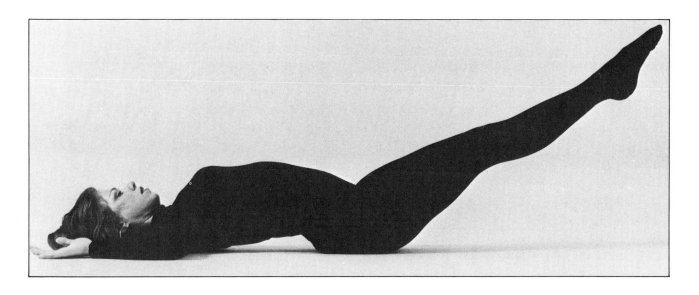

Performing the lifts this way requires an already well-conditioned set of stomach muscles, which is why I recommend that beginners and intermediates don't even attempt leg-ups. Instead, I recommend doing "leg-downs." Both legs are straightened to the ceiling at a 90-degree angle to the floor. Now, very slowly, lower your legs toward the floor without letting your lower back arch. At the moment your back wants to lose contact with the floor, stop and hold the leg position for 8 counts, then raise them up again. You may only be able to lower your legs a few inches before your back starts to arch. Fine. The important point is to keep your back flat on the floor and your stomach drawn in at all times. Repeat the "leg-downs" very slowly for as many times as your strength and ability permits. Doing the exercise this correct way is much more difficult for your stomach, and much more effective!

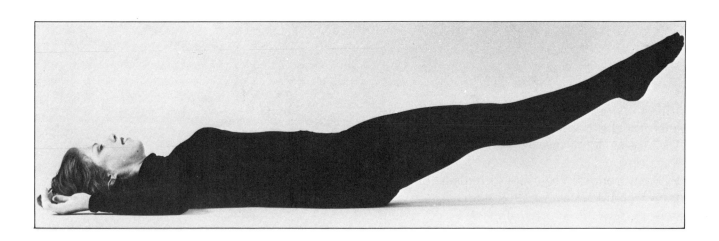

Sit-ups

Sit-ups may be the answer, for people who want to flatten their stomachs.

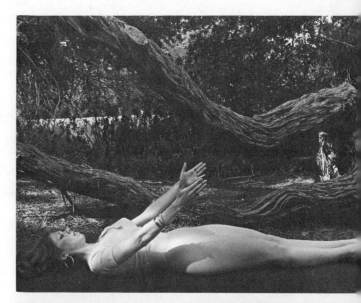

Position: Lie flat on your back with legs together and toes pointed. The stomach should be drawn in so that the lower back touches the floor. Arms are raised slightly.

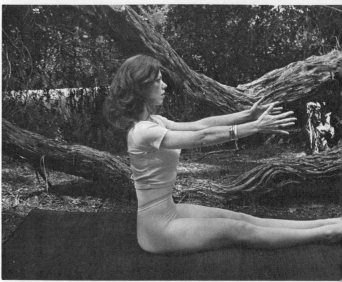

Beginners: Stretch your arms up and toward the toes while sitting up slowly (4 counts). Keep the back straight. Slowly lie back down (4 counts), still keeping the back straight, but stop at the third count. *Hold* for 4 more counts before continuing to the floor. Repeat for as long as your stamina will permit.

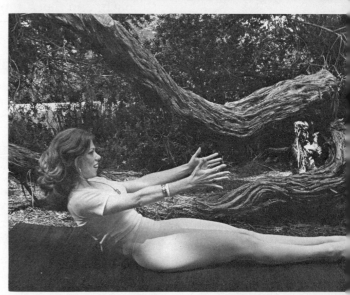

Intermediates: As you do the sit-ups, fold arms against the chest and grasp the elbows.

Advanced: Do sit-ups with arms extended out to the sides.

Body Awareness: Legs should remain together and feet should stay on the floor during this exercise. Draw the stomach muscles in or you'll be training them to pop out. Can you feel the upper abdomen muscles working?

Curl-ups

If you have dreams of strengthening a weak or bulging stomach, you'll want to seriously consider doing this classic, effective abdominal exercise every day. Unlike other sit-up exercises, this one emphasizes control, so don't rush your counts.

Position: Lie with your knees bent up and together. Feet are flat on the floor; arms folded in front.

Body Awareness: Try not to let your stomach pop out. Concentrate on pulling it in constantly. The feet should be touching the floor and the arms touching the body, or you're cheating. Are you feeling the abdominal muscles working for you?

Beginners: Place your feet farther from your buttocks, or anchor them in the opening under heavy furniture. Take 4 counts to curl straight up like a caterpillar, then lower again to the floor in 4 slow counts. As you lower, be sure you are curling down with the lower back touching the floor before the upper back.

Intermediates and Advanced: Bring your feet closer to the buttocks. Without anchoring your feet under furniture, do the beginner exercise. As you lower your back to the floor, stop halfway down (when just the lower back touches the floor, and hold the halfway position for eight counts. Repeat 4–12 times or as long as stamina permits.

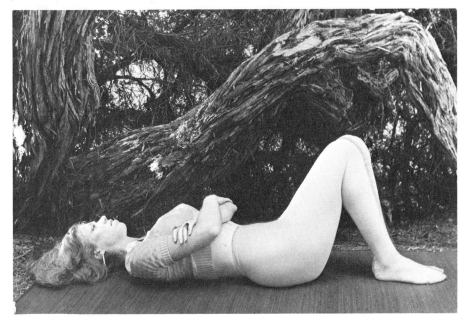

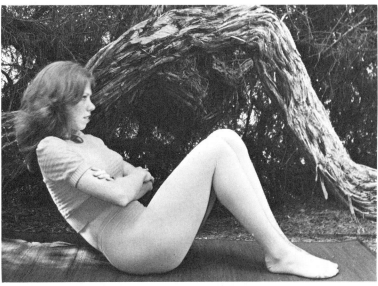

Gather-ups

Many people who ask me for help with a bulging midriff lament that they've tried doing sit-ups for years with little or no noticeable results. If you're one who feels discouraged about the results of your daily sit-up ritual, you might consider switching to this different and very effective stomach toner.

Position: Lie on your back with legs together and extended and arms reaching overhead on the floor.

Beginners and Intermediates: In one count, curl up by bringing the knees up and wrapping your arms around them. Your upper and lower body is gathered together in the middle, and you're balancing on your buttocks. Now the fun starts. From here, take 10 *very slow* counts to curl your way back to the floor. While your legs begin to straighten and lower toward the floor, your upper body is curling down: lower back, upper back, shoulders, neck, then head. The arms are reaching forward. Repeat the entire exercise 5–15 times, depending on stamina. Try not to rush your counts!

Advanced: Follow the above exercise, but add this one little move. When you curl your way back down to the floor, stop about halfway. Your lower legs should be parallel to the floor, knees still bent up. In this position, with your legs still in mid-air, bounce-rock by straightening and bending the knees out in front of you for 10 counts. Then curl all the way down to the floor. Repeat this version 5 or more times, depending on the stamina of the abdominal muscles.

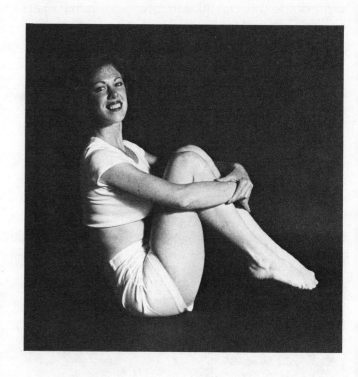

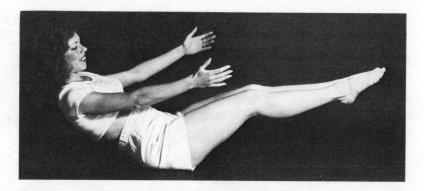

Body Awareness: To extract maximum benefit from this exercise, you'll need to be constantly drawing your stomach in, especially while you curl down. I'm sure you'll discover this exercise to be effective, especially if you supplement it by frequently holding in your stomach during the day!

Jackknife Sit-ups

These take less time than sit-ups to produce an effect.

Position: Lie on your back, arms stretched out to the sides, legs held tightly together, toes pointed, and stomach pressed in.

Beginners: In one fell swoop, boost your legs up as you simultaneously hoist your upper torso off the floor and throw your arms forward. You should be balancing on your buttocks, with legs and back about 6 inches off the floor. Relax down in 4 counts. Repeat 3 or more times in succession until stamina is depleted. Strive for a higher lift off the floor and an increase in the number of repetitions you perform.

Intermediates: Perform the beginner exercise 4 times. For the next 4 sit-ups, boost yourself higher up, then hold the jackknife pose for 4 counts before relaxing to the floor.

Advanced: Start with the beginner, then the intermediate sets. For the third set, try to touch your hands to feet as you balance—hold for 4–6 counts each time.

Body Awareness: You will not be able to balance if your back is rounded or if the legs and back are unequal distances from the floor (if the legs are higher, expect to roll backward). I remind my students to contract their stomach just before doing the sit-up, or else they defeat the purpose of the exercise.

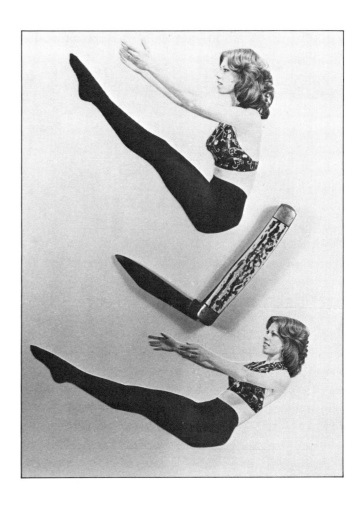

Contraction Sit-ups

> CAUTION: **Not for people with low-back problems.**

A more strenuous sit-up for a strong, supple back and a toned abdomen).

Position: Lie on your back with legs together, toes pointed, and arms extended diagonally overhead on the floor.

Beginners: In 4 counts, arch your back off the floor, dropping your head back. The top of your head and your hands stay on the floor, and you are looking upside down. (Feel the neck muscles stretching?) Hold for 2 counts, then slide your back down to the floor, and relax for 4. Repeat 4–6 times.

Intermediates: Start with the beginner version and continue arching your back and dropping your head until you come to a sitting position. Let the hands trail on the floor behind you as you arch up. When you arrive at a full sit, begin to curl back down to the floor for 4 counts with your arms reaching forward. Repeat 4–6 times in succession, slowly undulating as you arch up and curl down.

Advanced: Follow the intermediates by arching

all the way up. Then whip the arms forward, bringing your chest to your thighs. Stretch into your legs for 4 counts, then curl back down to the floor in 4 counts. Relax and repeat at least 3 more times. The 4-count arch, whip-forward, stretch, and curl-down should be a continuous flow without a pause.

Body Awareness: Try for the greatest back-arch possible by drawing the shoulder blades together and leading up with the chest. As you curl down, contract the stomach muscles. Feel the back, stomach, and leg muscles working?

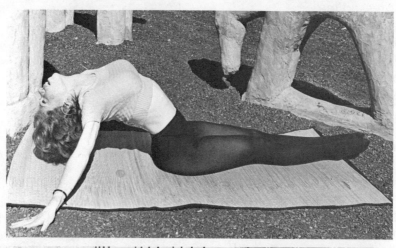

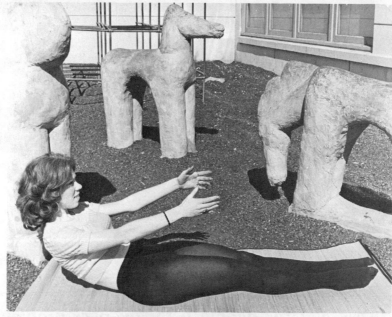

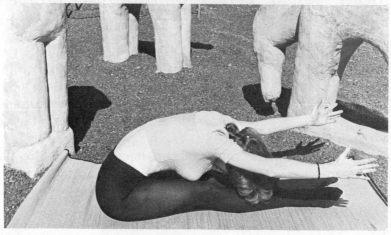

Leg-drops

This exercise is doubly effective, since it strengthens the stomach and tones the thigh muscles simultaneously.

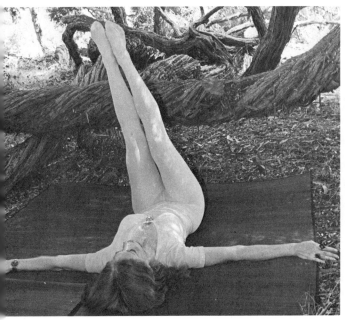 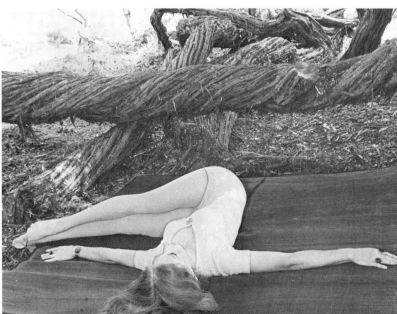

Position: Lie on your back with arms extended to the sides. Your legs should be together and lifted straight up.

Beginners: Bend your knees slightly. Lower both your legs to the right, trying to touch your toes to the right hand (4 slow counts to lower). Just touch the floor slightly. If you let your legs come crashing down, you'll have a hard time lifting them up again! Raise the legs up slowly (4 counts) and continue to the left side. Repeat the set at least 3 times.

Intermediates and Advanced: Keep your legs completely straight and point your toes. Try the set 4 times or more.

Body Awareness: Keep the legs glued together, especially when lifting them. Let your stomach do the work by pulling it in as you lower and lift your legs. Can you feel the muscles in your stomach and thighs toning?

Curl-downs

Here's a serious toner for weak or bulging abdomens.

Position: Sit with your knees bent up and feet together on the floor close to your buttocks. Stretch your arms forward, and pull your stomach in hard.

Beginners: In 4 *slow* counts, curl backward until your lower back touches the floor but your upper back is off the floor. Hold the curled position for 8 slow counts, then straighten up again in 4 counts. Repeat the exercise 4–8 times in succession. Pause for a few seconds, then repeat for another set of 8, or as many times as stamina permits.

If you're having difficulty keeping your feet on the floor when you curl down, you can hook them under a heavy piece of furniture. Later, try to perform the exercise without the aid of the furniture's weight.

Intermediates: After you've curled down to your lower back, raise one leg straight up in the air. Flex the foot by pushing through your heel. Hold the position for 8 counts. Now curl up in 4 counts, keeping the leg high in the air (keep smiling)! Return to starting position and continue the exercise 8 times in succession, alternating legs. Relax, then perform another round of 8.

Advanced: Curl down until your lower back touches the floor. Now straighten *both* legs in the air and hold the position 6–8 counts. Curl up while the legs remain in the air. Return to starting position and continue the exercise 6–8 times without pausing. Relax, then repeat another set of 6, or as many as stamina permits.

Body Awareness: As you curl down, concentrate on pulling in your stomach and keeping the shoulders relaxed. If you let them bunch up you'll create neck strain. Some of my students find it helpful, at first, to cushion the tail bone. As the stomach and hip muscles become stronger, you should be able to curl back so you are not positioned directly on your tail bone. Do you feel those abdominals building strength?

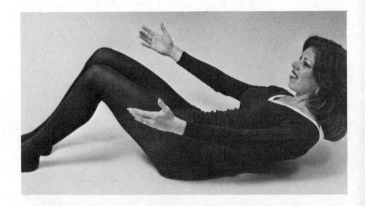

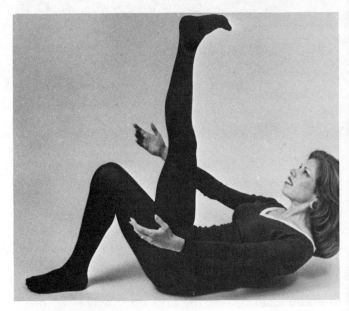

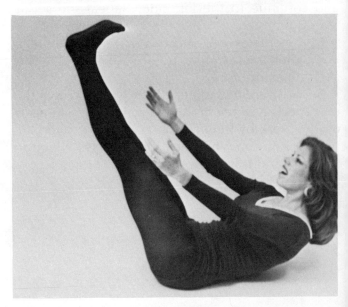

The Technique: Waist-Abdominal Stretches

Pretzel Twist

The Pretzel Twist is a twister that gives the body a good, all-around stretch, especially for your waist and back.

1. Sit with the right leg folded in front, the heel under the left thigh.

2. Cross the left leg over the right with the knee up and the left foot flat on the floor and close to the right knee.

3. The left buttock will want to come up, but force it down and straighten the back.

4. Place the left hand behind you on the floor.

5. Put the right elbow into the side of the left knee.

6. Now push the left knee to the right with the elbow as you twist around to the left. Twist as far as possible and hold for 8 counts.

7. Relax and repeat the twist 2 more times without leaving the position.

8. If you got into this position, you can get out of it and change sides!

Body Awareness: Work at keeping both buttocks on the floor and the back straight. Feel the muscles in the buttocks, waist, and back stretch.

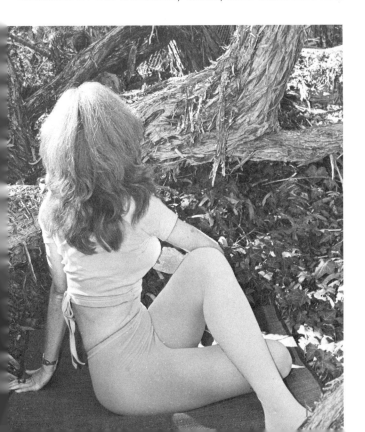
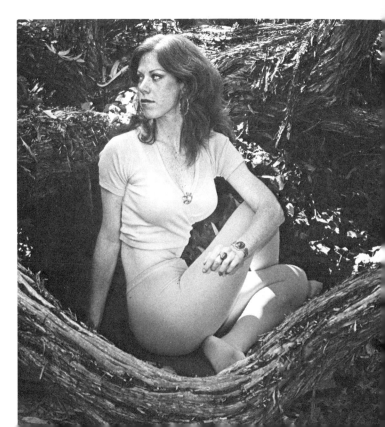

Seated Rib-Cage Isolation

A sway to trim your waistline.

Position: Sit with your feet crossed in front of you. Elongate your back and flatten your abdomen. Press your shoulder tips down and keep them relaxed.

Beginners: Place your hands on the knees. Take 4 counts to shift your rib cage only as far to the right as it will reach. Don't let your left buttock come off the floor, and try not to move your shoulders. Hold for 4 counts. Then shift the rib cage to the left and hold your position. Continue shifting and swaying (and holding) from side to side for 8 or more times in succession. Relax, then repeat the set.

Intermediates: Open your arms to the sides and shift the rib cage to the right (4 counts). Now bounce-reach the rib cage to the right 4 times. You should feel a stretch along the left side. Shift the ribs left and repeat. Continue for 6–8 times, alternating sides. Relax, then repeat the set.

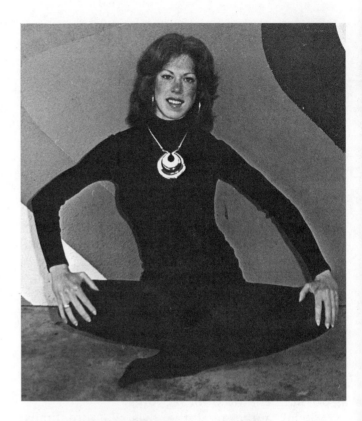

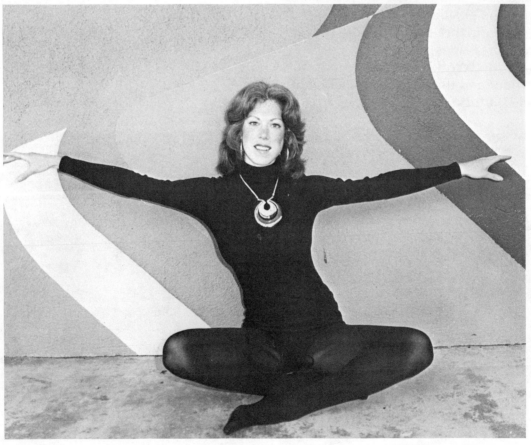

Advanced: Stretch your arms overhead and press shoulder tips down. Reach up to the ceiling 8 times, alternating arms. Keeping your arms overhead, shift the rib cage only from side to side at least 8 times. Relax and repeat several times.

Body Awareness: Since you are isolating the movement in the waist area only, try not to move other parts of your body. Do you feel muscles in the waist and abdominal area stretching?

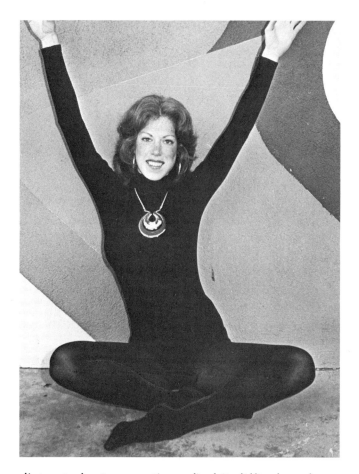

Standing Rib-Cage Isolations

A shifty way to whittle the waist: You can trim the waist and tone the upper arms by shifting your rib cage.

Position: Sit squarely on the edge of a chair with your back straight and stomach flattened. Stretch your arms sideways and lift your chest.

Beginners: Shift only your rib cage as far to the right side as it will stretch without moving your hips or shoulders. Now pulsate the rib cage over to the right side 8 times, keeping the shoulders level. Continue by shifting and bouncing it left for eight. Return to the right side for 4 bounces, then left for 4; then for 2 bounces each side, and finally alternate, in 1 count, from side to side several times so you are swaying from your midsection only. Relax a moment, then repeat the set twice more.

Intermediates: Stand with your feet wide apart. Squeeze your buttocks tightly together and stretch your arms sideways. Now follow the beginner exercise while standing.

Advanced: Perform one intermediate set. For the next 2 sets, stretch your arms overhead. As you shift and bounce the rib cage from side to side, keep the arms up high.

Body Awareness: My beginning and interme-

diate students sometimes find it difficult to keep the hips quiet while bouncing the rib cage. You can prevent them from moving by gripping the buttocks tightly together. You may find it helpful to perform the exercise in front of a mirror as you try to confine the movement to just the rib cage and waist. Are you feeling the stomach, waist, and arms toning?

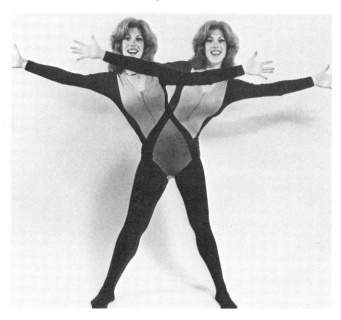

Seated Accordion

I've designed this long side-stretching exercise for anyone with unwanted waistline bulges.

Beginners: Sit on the right buttock with legs folded together to the left side. Place the left hand on the floor next to your knees. Reaching the right arm up and over toward the left side, bounce to the left 12 or more times. You will feel a greater stretch in the waist if the elbow doesn't bend while you are reaching and bouncing. Change sides so that the legs are bent to the right and you are sitting on the left buttock. Bounce 12 times to the right, then repeat the sequence.

Intermediates: Side-sit so that the right leg folds in front of you (heel to crotch) and the left leg folds to the side (heel to buttock). Try to keep both knees and both buttocks on the floor. Straighten your back. Bounce 12 times to the right, then to the left side, with one arm stretching overhead past the ear.

Advanced: Sit in a half side-split: one leg extends straight out to the side, toe pointed, the other leg is bent, heel touching the buttock. Try to feel the inner thigh muscles stretching as you take this position. Bounce to the right and left sides 12 times each, reaching one arm overhead past the ear as you bounce. Repeat the set.

Body Awareness: Draw the stomach in while you bounce. For maximum stretch benefit to the waist, try to bounce sideways without letting the chest twist forward. Feel as though the ribs are stretching apart like folds of an accordion.

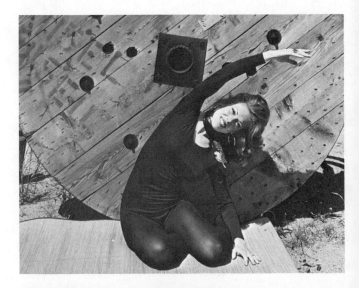

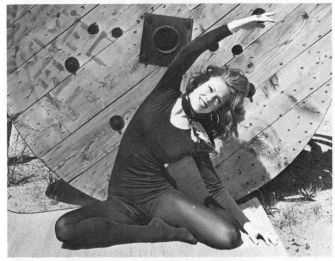

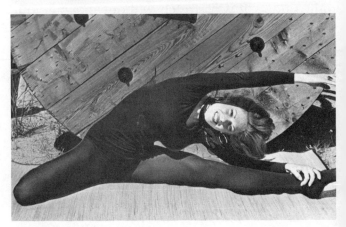

The Sidewinder

To diminish the waist and strengthen the arms.

Position: Stand with feet farther than shoulder-width apart, toes parallel and knees straight.

Beginners: Facing forward, slide the right arm down the side of the right leg to the knee. Meanwhile, reach the left arm overhead straight past the ear. Try to bend sideways as low as possible without twisting the hips or upper torso forward. Hold the sidestretch at your lowest possible stretch point for 8 counts, then come up and change sides. Repeat at least twice more.

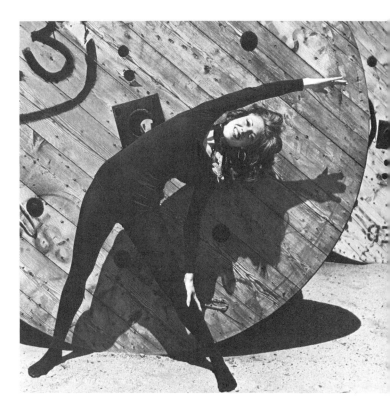

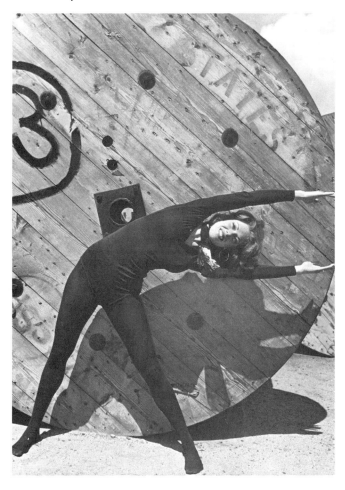

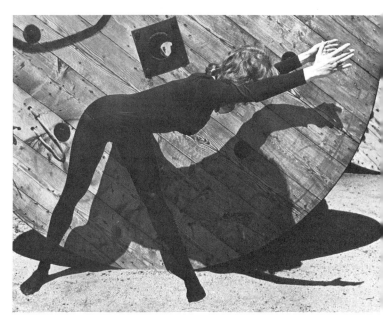

Intermediates: Follow the beginner exercise, but extend *both* arms out parallel (like railroad tracks), stretching them past the ears. Take 4 counts to bend sideways with arms extended. When you've reached your lowest stretch point, hold for 6 counts before returning upright. Repeat on the other side, then try each side again.

Advanced: Stretch sideways and hold for 6 counts as in the intermediate version. Instead of returning upright, roll the back out flat, paralleling it to the floor (chest facing the floor). Without letting the arms drop below ear level, hold the roll-out position for 4 counts. From there, return to the sideways stretch. Use 4 counts to straighten up, then begin stretching on the other side. Repeat the set once more on each side.

Body Awareness: You can avoid twisting the hips by pinching the buttocks together when you stretch sideways. Keep the shoulders down. For the greatest waist stretch, don't let the stomach pop out or the upper body cave in and collapse.

Windmill Lunge

This luxurious stretch trims the waistline while it tones your upper arms.

Position: Stand with your feet wide apart and toes parallel. Draw your stomach in and elongate your back. Bend just the right knee (the left one is straight).

Beginners: Reach your right arm overhead. For 8 counts bounce your knee down as you stretch your arm up. Feel the ribs separate along your right waistline from this opposition pull. Keep the elbow straight. Change arms and knees (bend the left knee, straighten the right) and repeat by stretching the left arm up while bending left knee for eight. Continue alternating sides for 8 counts (each side), then 4 counts, 2, and 1 count. Relax. Try the sequence again.

Intermediates: Perform the beginner sequence once. Then alter the position so you are bending the right knee and leaning your upper torso to the left. Now stretch your right arm overhead to the left side. Extend the left arm across your body. Follow the beginner exercise in this position (Bounce 8 times, then change sides for 8, 4, 2, and 1 count per side). Relax, then repeat the sequence.

Advanced: Try the intermediate sequence once. Now alter the position by bending the right knee and leaning upper torso to the left. Parallel both arms out to the left side and keep them close to the ears. Bounce-stretch to the left 8 times, then change sides and knees. Continue for 8, 4, 2, and 1 count each side. Repeat the sequence.

Body Awareness: Try to increase the range of each stretch impulse as you bounce and reach. You should be feeling the stretch impulse from the hip up through the fingertips. Do you also feel the upper-arm muscles building strength while your ribs separate as you reach?

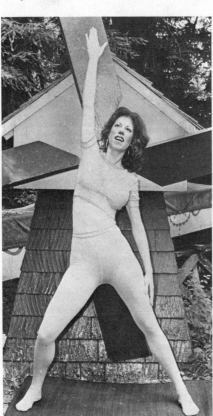 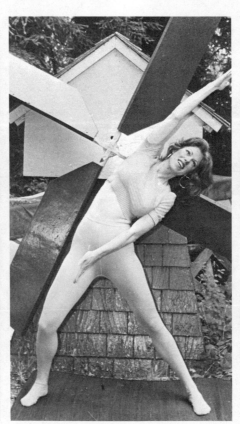 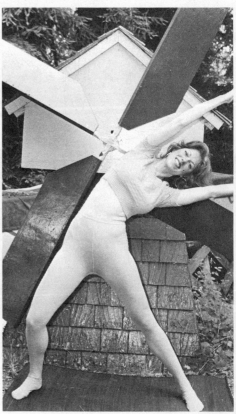

Roof-Plié Reach

Here's a split-level stretch that decreases your girth while you grow taller.

Position: Place your feet a little wider than shoulder-width apart, with toes turned out slightly. Draw your stomach in and extend your arms overhead next to your ears with your elbows kept very straight. Keep your head straight.

1. Reach one hand, then the other skyward, palms turned upward, as if you were trying to pick fruit from a high branch. Feel yourself growing out of your hips as you reach higher and higher for 16 counts. For a greater sense of upward expansion, press onto tiptoes and continue to stretch each arm higher and higher for 8 counts, palm up, as if you were pushing through the roof.

2. Without pausing, take 8 counts to bend the knees over the toes as you continue to stretch the arms skyward. Alternate parts 1 and 2 for 4 sets. Lower your arms for a moment, then repeat for 4 more sets.

Body Awareness: When you bend your knees, don't let your arms or chest collapse. Instead, lift your weight off of your knees by growing out of your hips. Be sure your stomach is flat, chest lifted, and rear tucked under slightly. Are you feeling your arms and thighs building strength while your midriff diminishes?

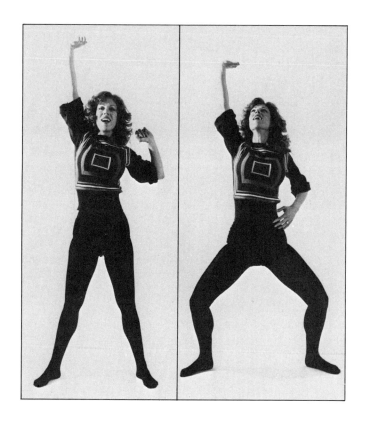

Secret Stomach Exercises (in public and private places)

● Pull your stomach in whenever you're awake. Think stomach and contract those muscles, especially when you:

brush your teeth	reach for anything
shower	wait for an elevator
shave	watch TV
dress	talk on the phone
cook	sit in the car.

● Try walking one block with the stomach drawn in, then one with it relaxed. Increase the number of blocks you hold it in.

● When bending your knees to pick up a heavy object, contract the stomach muscles. You'll notice that when you enlist the stomach muscles, the load is easier to lift.

● Deliberately put some frequently used objects on a high shelf so you are compelled to reach long through the waist to recover the items. Think of high shelving as a boon to the waist.

CHAPTER TWO:

HOW TO FIRM YOUR FANNY (TUSHY-TRIMMERS TO WORK YOUR BUTTOCKS OFF)

As humans, we stake claim to about 640 skeletal muscles of various sizes and shapes, and of all these muscles, the most massive, the heaviest (and potentially the strongest) is . . . you guessed it, the gluteus maximus, better known as the buttocks. Most of us think of our buttocks as protective padding to perch upon. But a muscle of such prodigious proportions surely has a more important function than merely soft cushioning for our sitting bones! Round, firm, fully packed buttock muscles are a real source of solid energy. As prime movers, the buttocks boost our bodies up inclines, provide the propulsion for running and walking, and help to extend and rotate the thighs. They're the main thrust in getting us up on our feet from a sitting position. Firm buttocks serve to buttress the lower back and to stabilize the hips and pelvis. If these all-powerful muscles are permitted to fall prey to sedentation, they turn into a very unappetizing mass of unrendered lard! Call it cellulite, call it fat, call it the cottage-cheese syndrome—a melting, sedentary, soft seat will broaden your backside and spoil your entire figure or physique. Weak, flabby buttock muscles can eventually instigate low-back pain and faulty leg alignment.

Like the buttocks, your hips are more than a resting place for your hands. The hips function to give strength, support, balance, force, and direction during locomotion. Walking actually initiates at the hip joint, not at the knee. The hips are the real control center from which all our body parts radiate outward. If the muscles around the hip joint (buttocks, thighs, and lower back) are strong, the pelvis can be kept steady and our balance is improved. But if the surrounding muscles are weak, the pelvis will tilt forward and downward, allowing all the abdominal contents (intestines, stomach, etc.) to spill forward and form a precariously hanging bulge. Whenever the front bulges, the rear protrudes.

Aside from causing an unstable pelvis, hip and buttock muscles that are allowed to weaken from too much sitting begin to grow "flab pockets" that can droop down along the sides of the upper thighs.

Women tend to accumulate fatty deposits along their upper thighs and buttocks, and to tone this area takes considerable, consistent effort! We can't alter our basic bone structure underlying the hips. Women inherit broader pelvic bones than men, and no amount of exercise can transform that basic bone structure. But specific exercises *can* remove cottage-cheese buttocks and saddlebags along the sides that make one look like a mail carrier for the Pony Express. So let's begin by thinking of the fanny as muscle to be firmed rather than padding on which to spread ourselves.

Select any or all of the exercises in this volume and do at least three *every day*, varying them whenever you like. You can't overdo it when it comes to fanny-firming, so get off your butt and let's get moving!

The Technique

Payoff Kickback

Kickbacks were designed especially to improve the tone of the buttock muscles and to give you a thigh stretch at the same time.

Position: Get down on all fours and extend the right leg straight back so that the pointed toe touches the floor. Keep you head level.

Beginners: Kick the right leg up high behind you and drop it to starting position 8 times in a row on the right side. Then bend the knee to your head as you round over and return to all fours. Repeat on the left side 3 more times before stopping. Each time you kick, lift your head and chest up high so that your back arches slightly.

Intermediates: With every kick, hold the leg up at its highest point for 4 counts before lowering. Kick, hold, and lower the leg 6 times before changing sides. Repeat without pausing.

Advanced: Same as intermediates, only double the number of kicks per side.

Body Awareness: Each kick shows a long, high, straight leg, not a bent knee. Those hips want to twist and turn sideways with every kick, but don't let them. If you keep your hips looking forward, you'll really feel the upper thigh and buttock muscles working!

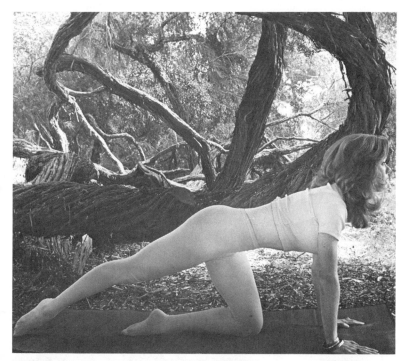

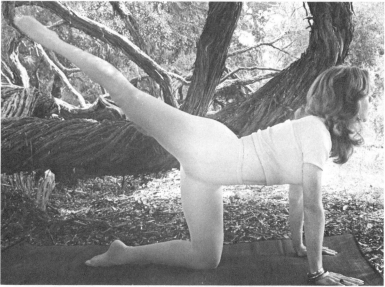

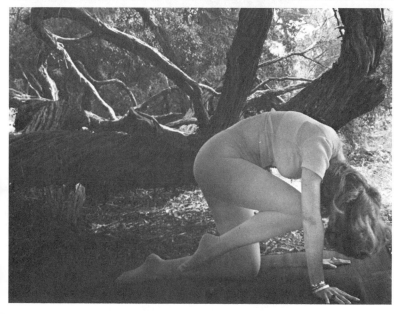

Rover's Revenge

This exercise helps reduce the flab pockets in the upper thighs and buttocks that drive women, in particular, crazy.

Position: On all fours, head up.

Beginners: (Cushion knees.) Raise one thigh to the side as high as possible with the knee bent, so you feel a stretch along the inner thighs. Straighten the leg out to the side without letting it drop in height. Hold it out for 4 beats, then bend it in and return it to the floor. Change legs. Repeat on both sides at least 3 more times.

Intermediates: After the leg is extended to the side, describe 8 small circles with the leg circling forward, then back for 4 counts. Bend the leg in, lower it, and change sides. Repeat at least once.

Advanced: Increase the circles to 32—8 forward, 8 back, 8 forward and 8 back, without pausing. Repeat the set on the other side.

Body Awareness: Try not to let the leg drop in height when circling it. Pointing the toes will help to straighten the working leg. Do you feel the muscles in *both* buttocks and upper thighs strengthening simultaneously?

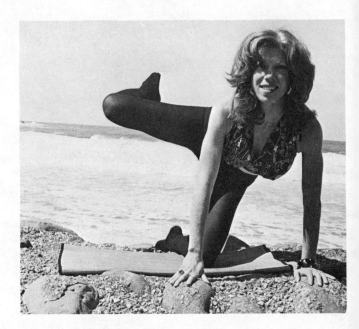

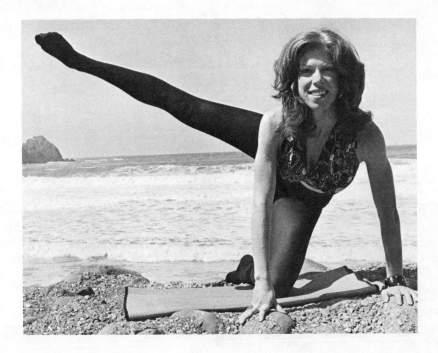

Rover's Sidekick

Solidifying sedentary spread: Little-used buttock and upper-thigh mucles turn to jelly and spread. Here's one way to tone them.

Position: Get down on all fours. Straighten your elbows and flatten your back so it is parallel to the floor. Keep your head up.

Beginners: Lift one thigh high to the side and hold it up for 4–8 counts without letting it drop. Now straighten the leg completely to the side, point the toes, and hold the leg out for another 4–8 counts. Be sure that your knee is straight. Bend the knee again and lower your leg to the floor. Repeat, then change sides. Continue the exercise for 8–10 times, alternating legs after every second set.

Intermediates: Lift one thigh to the side and hold it up for 2 counts. Straighten the leg sideways and hold it for 2 more counts. Now pulsate your leg up and down (little kicks) for 8–12 times while the leg is out to the side. Keep your kicking leg very straight, and don't let it drift backward while you kick. Set the leg down, then immediately change sides. Continue the exercise 6–8 times, alternating legs.

Advanced: Follow the intermediate version. After the leg pulsates 8–16 times in the air, hold it sideways and sit back onto the heel of your opposite foot. Hold-sit for 4–8 counts, then lean forward again (hands on the floor), and return to starting position. Change legs and continue the exercise 6–8 times, alternating legs.

Body Awareness: You're cheating if you let your elbows bend, or if your knee bends while the leg is kicking sideways. My beginning students usually feel buttock or hip cramps when they first try this exercise. I recommend lowering the leg and pounding or kneading the cramp with both hands. The cramp should subside quickly, and you can start all over again. The more often you perform this exercise, the less often you'll cramp.

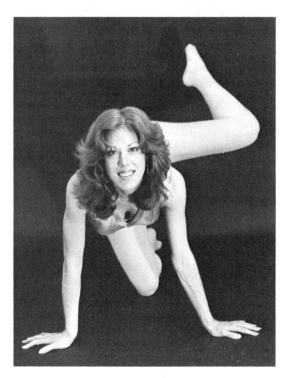
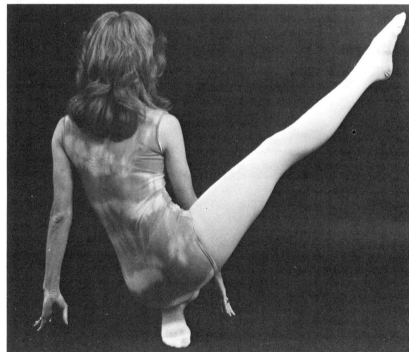

The Standing Sidekick

This and the next exercise will help firm the buttocks and upper thighs while you limber your back.

Position: Stand with your hands pressing a wall at shoulder level. Elbows are straight and your back is flat and parallel to the floor. Bring the feet together and straighten the knees.

Beginners: Raise the right leg directly sideways as high as possible for 4 counts. Try not to bend either knee. Point the right toes as you hold the leg in the air for 4–6 counts. Now lower it on 4 counts. Repeat on the left side. Continue the set for 4–6 times, alternating legs.

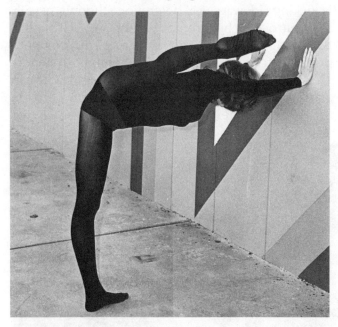

Intermediates: Follow the beginner version and pulsate the leg up in the air for 4 beats. Hold it up for 4 more beats. Lower the leg on 4. Repeat with the other leg. Continue the set for 4 times, alternating legs. Relax, then repeat 4 more times.

Advanced: Stand with knees straight. Place the hands flat on the floor in front of the toes. Now raise the right leg directly sideways as high as possible. Hold it up for 4 counts. Beat it up for 4. Hold it up for another 4 counts. Lower the leg on 4. Change sides. Repeat the set 4–6 times, alternating legs.

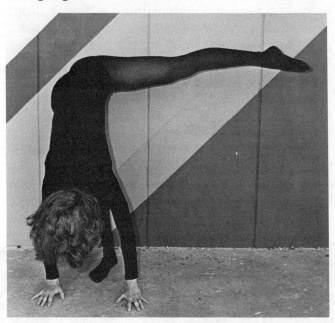

Body Awareness: Try to lengthen your back without tensing up your shoulders. If you are feeling a shin strain on the standing leg, then you are letting too much of your weight fall onto it. Try to center your weight evenly on both hands. Do you feel the buttock and thigh muscles firming as the leg and back muscles are stretching?

The Standing Kickback

Position: Stand arm's distance from a wall with your feet together and knees straight. Press both hands against the wall, shoulder level, with elbows straight. Your back should be flat and parallel to the floor, your head level with the back.

Beginners: Raise the right leg as high as possible directly behind you in 4 counts. Point the toes as you hold the leg up high for 6–8 counts without twisting your hips. Lower it on 4, and change sides. Continue the set for 6–8 times, alternating legs. Each time, try to raise your leg just a fraction higher.

Intermediates: Follow the beginner version. While the leg is in the air, pulsate it up for 4–6 beats. Hold it up 4 more beats. Now lower it on 4. Repeat, then change legs. Continue the set for 4–6 times, alternating legs every second set. Relax, then repeat 4 more sets.

Advanced: Stand with your knees straight and palms flat on the floor in front of the toes. Raise the right leg high behind you. Hold it up for 4 counts; beat it up for 4, splitting the legs apart. Hold it up for 4 more counts, then lower it on 4. Repeat the set, then change legs. Continue the set 4–6 times, changing legs every second set.

Body Awareness: You cheat if your knees or elbows bend. Your hips want to twist sideways when you kick, but try to keep the hip bones facing down and forward. Pointing the toes helps to straighten the kicking leg. Do you feel the thigh and buttock muscles toning as the leg and back muscles are stretching?

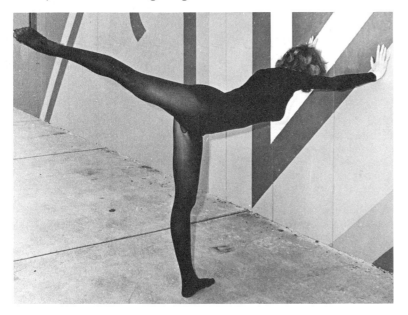

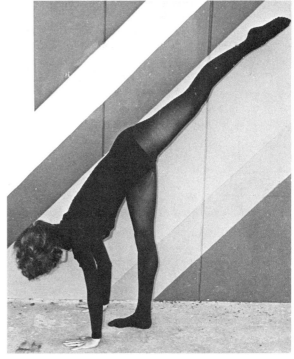

The Toad

I call this exercise the Toad, a three-for-the-effort-of-one exercise that will stretch and tone the buttocks, thighs, and long back muscles.

Position: Sit with your legs folded in front of you, keeping your right heel toward the crotch and the left heel against your right ankle. Try to flatten your knees to the floor and stretch your back.

Beginners: Place your hands on the floor in front of your knees. Keep your back flat and hold your head up; bend elbows as you lower your chest as close to the floor as you can. When you've lowered your chest as far as possible, hold for 8 counts. Now bounce gently 8 times toward the floor, keeping your back flat and your head up. Straighten up in 4 counts. Try to repeat the exercise 4 times without pausing; then change positions of legs and repeat 4 times.

Intermediates: Follow the beginner instructions, but place your forearms and elbows on the floor in front of your knees. Your head will drop lower. Try to keep your back as flat as possible.

Advanced: Warm up with one set of the intermediate exercise. Then place your arms and elbows on the floor, lowering your chest to your legs. Now try to place your right ear on the floor and hold for 4 counts, and reverse with the left ear. Straighten up on 4 and repeat. Change legs and do one intermediate version before performing two advanced exercises.

Body Awareness: If your buttocks lift off the floor, you're cheating. Keep your stomach pulled in, even while bouncing. Do you feel the stretch along your back, buttocks, and thighs?

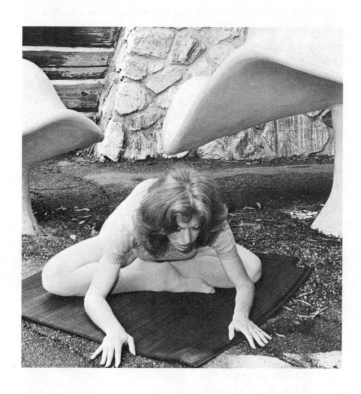
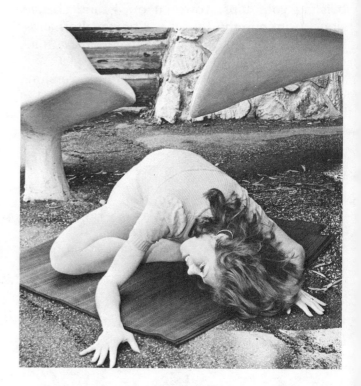

The Fish

CAUTION: **Check with your doctor first if you have a problem lower back.**

Tone up the buttocks and hips while strengthening the lower back.

Position: Lie face down with chin and shoulders on the floor. Point your toes and straighten the knees.

Beginners: Place your hands palms down alongside your thighs. Lift one leg high behind you without twisting your hips. Hold it up for 8 counts then lower it. Repeat with the other leg. While the leg is lifted, pulsate it up behind you 8 times. Alternate sets for 4–6 times.

Intermediates: Follow the beginners' version sets. For a third set, raise both legs together from the hip as high as possible and hold them up for 4–8 counts. Lower them, then repeat 3 sets twice or more without pausing.

Advanced: Alter the position so your arms extend straight forward and the chin is on the floor. In this position, follow the intermediate sets for 2–4 times.

Body Awareness: Try to raise the legs from your hips so that the thighs come off the floor. Your legs will lift higher if you supersqueeze your buttocks together, and if you try to keep your shoulders down. You're cheating if the knees bend.

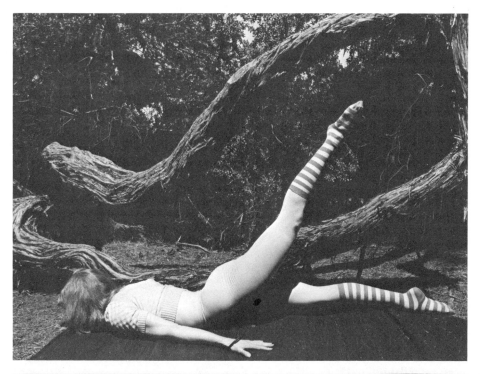

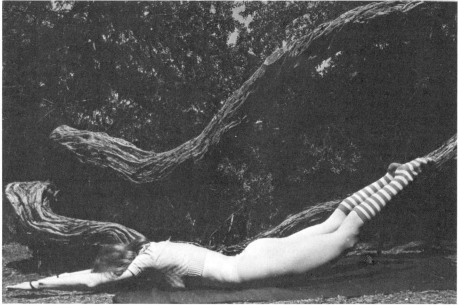

Fish with Chair

CAUTION: *If you have low-back problems, check with your doctor before trying this exercise.*

Typically, by heredity's design (or from lack of exercise), women wear their flesh around the buttocks, upper thighs, and upper arms; while men wear theirs around the midriff. This doesn't mean that your softwear can't be firmed, it only means that the soft spots require a variety of concentrated exercises. Here's one simple exercise that will help to firm up a baggy rear end.

Position: Lie on your stomach with your hands at your sides. Squeeze your two legs together as if they were one, and straighten the knees so they are not touching the floor. Grip your buttocks tightly together.

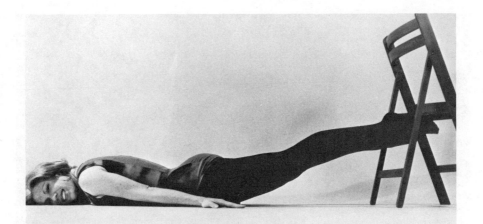

Start: With your legs glued together and your buttocks contracted, lift your feet, knees, and thighs off the ground. Press your feet ino the seat of the chair and hold for 8–16 counts, then lower the legs. Repeat the exercise 4 or more times in succession. Be sure you're gripping the muscles hard. Try the exercise again later in the day, as many times as possible.

Body Awareness: You're cheating if you let your knees bend or your legs separate. For best results, do the exercise daily, and become accustomed to really squeezing your buttock muscles.

The Foldout

Two hard-to-tone areas of the body are the buttocks and upper thighs. Here's one simple but effective exercise to get you started.

Position: Side-sit with right leg folded in front, heel to crotch, and left leg folded to the side, heel to buttock. Try to sit squarely on both buttocks. Lengthen your back. You may feel a stretch along the top of the left thigh in this position. Open arms to the sides.

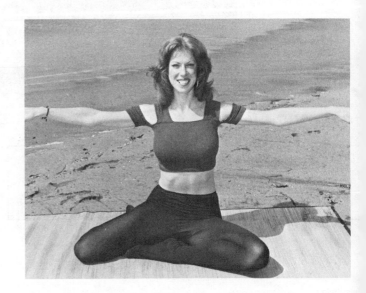

Beginners and intermediates: Raise just your left buttock off the floor and hold it up for 4 counts. Now raise the left leg off the floor a few inches (keep the knee bent) and hold it up for 4 slow beats. Lower the leg, and repeat 2 or 3 more times. Change sides so the left leg is bent in front and the right leg is folded to the side. Repeat on the second side twice. When you are in the side-sit position, both buttocks and both knees should be touching the floor.

Advanced: Lift the left leg off the floor a few inches and hold it up for 4 beats. Now straighten the left leg sideways in the air and hold it for 4 more counts. Keeping it straight, kick it up gently 4 times. Then fold it in on 4 counts, and set it down. Repeat the set twice more. Change sides for 3 sets.

Body Awareness: When you raise your left leg, try not to lean too far over to the right. Work at straightening your back. You may feel a cramp in the lifted buttock—a sign of muscle weakness from disuse. If a cramp occurs, set the leg down and pound out the cramp gently with your fists. As you practice this exercise more, cramps will decrease. Feel the buttock and upper-thigh muscles toning?

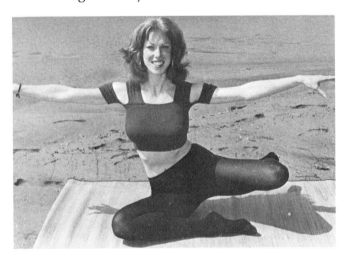
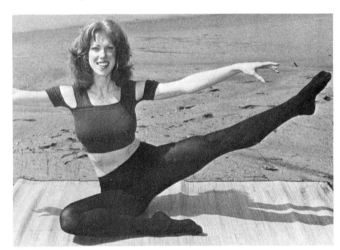

Swooping

A stretch for the buttocks, thighs, and back.

Position: Sit with the right leg folded in front, heel to crotch; left leg folded to the side, heel to buttock. Try to sit squarely on both buttocks with both knees on the floor. You may feel a thigh-stretch in this position, or you may find that the right knee won't stay on the floor. If so, let the knee come up until you develop more stretch along the front thighs. Lengthen your back.

Beginners: Stretch your arms back as you lean forward with a straight, flat back (no rounded shoulders). Bounce forward 8 times, aiming your chest to the floor but keeping your head up. Straighten up and relax a moment, then repeat 2–4 more times. The first set of bounces should be done slowly and gently, to warm up. Aim closer to the floor with each set, being careful not to strain. Change legs and repeat 2–4 times.

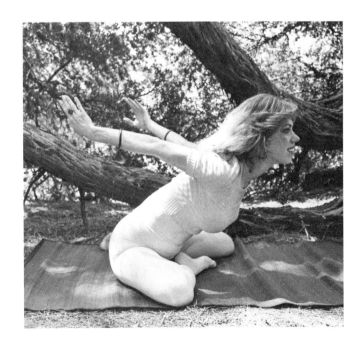

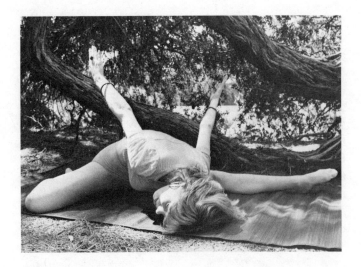

Intermediates: Follow the beginner exercise by bouncing forward 8 times. For the second and third set, try to touch your right, then left ear to the floor in front of you when you bounce.

Advanced: Alter the sitting position so that the right leg is extended sideways on the floor with toes pointed. The left leg remains folded, heel to buttock. Now follow the intermediate version in this half-split position, swooping forward for 8 times. Straighten up, then repeat, this time touching one ear to the floor. Change legs for 2 sets. Relax, then repeat the sequence. You should be feeling the inner-thigh muscles stretching as you swoop forward, but be careful not to overpull them!

Body Awareness: Concentrate on keeping your back very flat by drawing your shoulder blades together and your stomach in when you swoop forward. You're cheating if your shoulders round.

Karate Kick

For balance and buttocks. Having good balance is of key importance to performing any sport skillfully. Here's a kicking exercise borrowed from karate that lets you practice your balance while you tone your hips, upper thighs, and fanny.

Position: Stand sideways to a wall (or any support) and touch it with one hand. Raise the opposite leg sideways, to hip level, with your knee bent and foot flexed up. Your thigh should be parallel to the floor.

Beginners: Keep your leg at hip level and snap it bent, then straight, quickly for 16 animated counts. Put real power into each snap, especially when you straighten the knee. Change sides and repeat for 16. Try the exercise a second time.

Intermediates: Follow the beginner exercise without holding a wall or support. Let your arms drop by your sides. Your balance will improve if you try not to move any part of your body except the kicking leg that snaps bent and straight.

Advanced: Raise your thigh higher than hip level and lean slightly away from the raised leg. You can let your arms drop by your sides or position them in a karate block. Make a fist with both hands, bend one arm in front of your body, and straighten the other arm sideways toward your foot. Now snap the leg back and forth 16 times while you keep it higher than hip level.

You may lean away from the leg when you kick. Change sides and repeat. Try the exercise a second time.

Body Awareness: You're cheating if you let your knee drop in height during any part of the exercise! In this case, you can let both knees bend slightly at all times. Are you feeling those buttock and hip muscles toning and the inner thighs stretching?

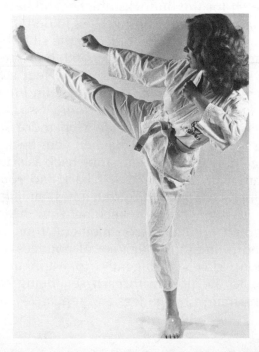

Sidesaddle Kick

Here's one exercise I've designed to tone and strengthen bulging "hip pockets," but you'll need to perform it daily if you want results.

Position: Lie on one side in a straight line. Prop your head up on one hand and place the other hand on the floor in front of your stomach. Point your toes.

Beginners: Kick your top leg up high and slightly backward, then lower it to meet the bottom leg. Repeat the kicking action for 16 snappy counts, concentrating on a high kick slightly behind your bottom leg. Rest, then repeat for another 16 counts. Now roll over onto your other side and repeat the exercise twice. When you improve, try to perform the exercise 3 times on one side before changing legs.

Intermediates: Perform the beginner exercise 3 times on one side. Now raise your top leg as high as possible and hold it up for 4 counts. Raise the bottom leg to meet it, and hold both legs up for 8 counts. Repeat this hold sequence, then roll over onto the other side and perform the entire exercise from the beginning.

Advanced: Perform the intermediate version on one side. While both legs are raised, keep them high and scissors-kick by alternating legs forward and backward for 8–16 counts. Repeat the entire sequence on the other side.

Body Awareness: For maximum benefit, draw your stomach in whenever you kick, and always kick slightly back. Keep your body lying in a straight line. Are you feeling your buttock and thigh muscles toning?

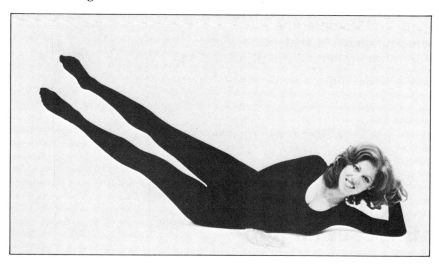

Hip-Shoulder Isolation

Have you noticed that some people move through life with the greatest of ease, grace, and fluid coordination, while others go about routine living looking loutish and stiff? The way a person moves—walks, stands, sits, gestures—can reveal the psychological state he or she has adopted. A loose, fluid, well-coordinated body often indicates a friendly, generous, optimistic personality in tune with self and open to others. A body that is stiff, lubberly, or uncoordinated can indicate a more stubborn, tense, less-integrated personality. It's no secret that when you learn how to free your body and skillfully coordinate your movements, you free your soul and become more in tune with your physical and emotional self.

Here is one simple exercise that challenges you to loosen (and coordinate) different parts of your body, especially your hips.

Position: Stand with your feet a little more than shoulder-width apart, with your weight placed evenly on both feet. Bend your knees slightly and place hands on hips.

Hips: Keeping your knees loose and slightly bent, throw one hip out to the side without shifting your weight. The shoulders don't move— only the hip that you've pushed out sideways.

Return to center, then push the other hip sideways without moving your shoulders. Continue shifting your hips only from side to side for a while. If you're getting good at this, try pushing the hips backward and forward without swaying your upper body back and forth. Try the hip moves to music of varied tempi. The idea is to get them swaying from side to side (then forward and back) without interference from the rest of your body.

Coordinate: While the left hip is thrown to the side, lift the right shoulder at the same time. Try that 4 times, then coordinate the movement 4 times on the other side (lift your left shoulder when pushing the right hip sideways). Repeat the coordinated hip-shoulder movements until they feel comfortable, then try alternating after every 2, then after each count.

Body Awareness: Expect this exercise to feel awkward at first. Once you get the knack of it (try it to music) you'll begin to feel your hips and shoulders loosening up and coordinating with less concentration on your part. At that point, really exaggerate the movements and let the hips and shoulders move to the extreme.

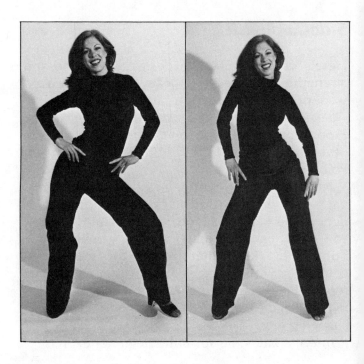

Secret Fanny Exercises (in public and private places)

If you're firmly committed to your fanny, you should incorporate the following habits during the day to augment your exercise time. Here are a few ideas to get you started. Have fun!

● Instead of using your hands, squeeze your buttock and upper-thigh muscles together to lift off of a chair.

● The reverse also applies—pinch the buttocks together *before* sitting in a chair.

● When you shake someone's hand, press your buttocks together and hold. Release the contraction when you release hands.

● When the phone rings, contract your buttocks as you stand up and reach for it. Whenever the caller speaks, squeeze and hold the contraction. Release when *you* speak.

● While you are standing—brushing your teeth, waiting in a line, doing dishes, cooking, etc.— imagine that you have a precious coin between your buttocks and you cannot drop it!

● While in a long meeting or at a double feature, occasionally contract and hold the buttocks together to keep the muscles from going numb.

● Practice walking briskly a few blocks while you forcibly tighten each buttock so that you feel your strides all the way up to your hips.

● While sitting on a bus or at your desk, press your legs and buttocks tightly together and hold a few seconds (or longer). Alternate contracting with relaxing.

CHAPTER THREE:

HOW TO BANISH BACKACHES

It all started with 28 inches. It seems so simplistic to us now, just a slight shift of 28 inches from a horizontal to a vertical position, and we became lords over all other living creatures. The direction of our 28-inch undulating caterpillar-shaped support has been one of the most profound and important evolutionary developments. When we became bipeds, we freed our hands to become the servants of our minds. All the heavy supporting that our hands bore was taken up by the feet and the now-vertical column. Man's brain became the guide of his freed hands, while the spine became the real backbone of his evolved achievements.

The spine has 24 movable bones (vertebrae) separated by 23 spongy, flexible discs (cartilage) that look like jelly doughnuts. Their profile forms a long S-shaped curve with three gentle slopes: one indented curve at the back of the neck, another at the lower back, and an outward curve at the upper back. These graceful curves make the spine 16 times stronger and more capable of bearing weight than if it were completely straight. The long, thin tube is held together by ligaments and is supported on all sides by muscles that run like cables up the back, along the sides, in the front (abdominal muscles), and at the base (buttock and hip muscles). It is these muscles surrounding and supporting all sides of the spine that give the column its ability to stabilize the upper body.

The curves in your spine, although not as alluring as the curves elsewhere in the body, are the most important ones structurally. Their degree of roundedness or flatness can predict the condition of the surrounding muscles and your predisposition to back pain.

One day in your routine living you innocently bend down, or turn to the side, or reach overhead, and from out of nowhere, without warning, a bolt of "lightning" strikes you in the back. You are immediately immobilized, dazed, locked in agony. Your slightest attempt to straighten out triggers a piercing electric shock. You feel like a helpless cripple paralyzed by pain, praying that someone will come along with a stretcher.

Maybe this is your introduction to back pain, or maybe you were silently suffering from mild but nagging backaches prior to the acute attack. Regardless of its chronic or acute nature, once a back pain strikes, it will return repeatedly and intensely to squelch your zest for life unless you take the initiative to reeducate your muscles.

If, for example, the lower-back muscles are weak, the weight of your upper body will drop and settle down, making the lower back "sway" into an exaggerated bow. The cushioning discs in the low back are then compressed like limp springs in a saggy mattress, and create friction between the bony vertebrae, thereby pinching the nerves. We feel the crush as low-back pain.

The same indented sway can be due to slack stomach muscles. If the abdominal wall isn't strong enough to brace the contents within, then the heavy organs come spilling forward, coaxing the lower back to deepen its curve, to cave in, and to put pressure on the discs.

But if the buttock and hip muscles are firm, they can buttress the base of the spine and prevent the pelvis from tipping too far forward (another cause for a concave lower back).

The spinal slopes go through normal and abnormal changes in shape, depending on the posture we assume. Usually one excessive curve in the column throws the other two into excess. A hunched or rounded upper back is often accompanied by a poked crane neck and a concave (or convex) lower back.

When the spine's support muscles are stiff or flaccid, and when the posture we habitually assume tends to exaggerate the curves rather than to diminish them, we become easy victims of an epidemic that has inflicted our adult population to agonizing proportions: the backache, or the bad-back syndrome.

Most back problems are from slothful, slouchy posture that depresses the spine into a pile of sunken bones, placing stress and strain on the nerves, discs, ligaments, tendons, and support muscles. A person with good posture distributes forces and weights evenly along the spine. But a sloppy stance tends to localize a force or pressure in one area, predisposing that area of the back to pain and injury.

Since muscles are also affected by our emotions, the spine might slump like deflated folds of an accordion in reflection of a depressed, dejected mood. If we carry the weight of the world on our shoulders, we tend to slump. When we feel accomplished or attractive, the spine tends to straighten and expand in response.

Emotional stress can cause muscles to tense and contract as if to prevent further outside impingements. If the emotional conflict goes unresolved, aches from tense, stiff muscles are often felt as neck and back pain. A physical or psychological release can ease the muscle tension.

There are other reasons for back pain: disease, aging, pregnancy, physiological defects, referred pain from other parts of the body, etc. But for the majority, back pain is caused by slouching and by underexercised muscles due to sedentary living.

If you suffer from a bad back, you should consult your doctor before trying any of the exercises in this book. If you are swaybacked, try to avoid those particular exercises that arch the back (bending backward) until your stomach and buttock muscles are strong and the low-back curve show signs of diminishing. Your abdomen must equal or exceed the strength of your lower back if it is to be supportive.

After back pain diminishes, there is only one superior preventative: habitually adjusting your posture to keep the spine lengthened, and exercising the muscles daily (about 20 minutes). Back exercises are done to relieve pain *and* to prevent it from occurring. Only strong, supple spinal muscles can stabilize the backbone and free us from becoming prisoners of our own pain.

I've divided the back exercises in this chapter into three types. The first section consists of easier exercises for those with delicate backs. If you suffer from back problems, have your doctor select the exercises in this first section that he/she would best help alleviate your particular problem.

In the next section, "Back-Hamstring Connection," more extreme back-stretches are introduced for those with normal or improved backs who want to prevent pain by developing fabulous flexibility forever! You'll notice that exercises in this section have you stretching your hamstring muscles (behind your thighs) at the same time that you're stretching your back. These two sets of muscles work in concert. If your hamstrings are too stiff (i.e., you can't straighten out your legs completely) you won't be able to stretch your back very far. Likewise, if your back is too stiff, then your legs won't straighten completely. All of the exercises in this section give you wonderful opportunities gradually to develop super suppleness.

The last section consists of backward stretches, which also help to strengthen your lower back and shoulders while you're stretching the chest and neck muscles. Be careful—back bends are for people with *healthy* backs.

Since all of the exercises in this chapter also serve to help you release tension and promote relaxation, I know you're going to appreciate them. These are the luxurious stretches, so let yourself enjoy them!

The Technique: Gentle Forward Stretches for Delicate Backs

The Backslide

This stretch brings relief for low-back pain and helps to correct a swayback.

Position: Lie on a hard surface (not a cushy rug or bed). Bend the knees up and place the feet flat on the floor close to your buttocks. Arms may be at the sides or stretched out. Melt your back, neck, and shoulders into the floor. Shrink the stomach in, and let the hips tilt up slightly. Squeeze your buttock muscles together.

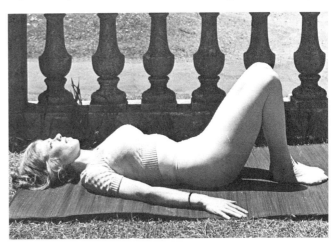

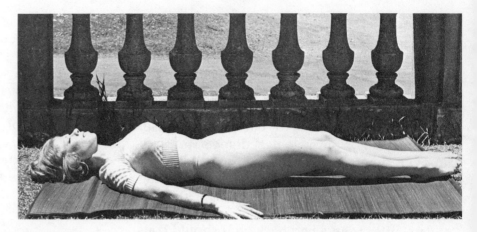

Start: Very slowly slide your feet forward along the floor for 8 counts. As your legs begin to straighten, the lower back or shoulders might try to sneak up off the floor; don't let them! Slide the legs only as far as your back and shoulders will remain on the floor. Hold for 8 counts. Then slide the feet up to the buttocks again and repeat. Try this exercise at least 3 times in succession, performing it as often during the day as you

desire. You are trying to straighten your legs completely while you keep the lower back, the shoulders, and the neck glued to the floor.

Body Awareness: To help push your back down, pull your abdominal muscles in. Constantly pinch the buttock muscles together, but relax the shoulder tips so they don't hunch up or round. This exercise should feel expecially good in the lower-back region.

The Backrest

To gently stretch the spine and tone the stomach muscles.

Position: Lie on your back with knees bent to the chest and feet together. Grasp the outside ankles. Shrink your stomach to the floor.

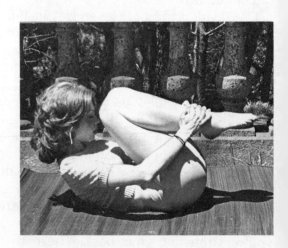

Beginners: As you pull your knees to your chest, raise your head and shoulders toward your knees in 4 counts. Bounce the head toward the knees for 4, then lower to the floor for 4. Repeat 4–6 times, keeping the legs together.

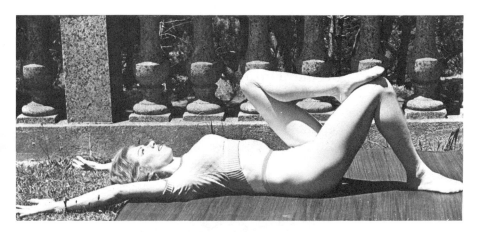

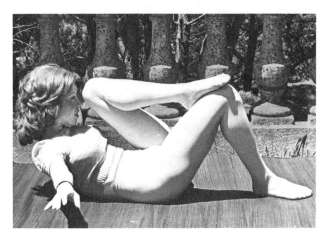

Intermediates: Alter the above position so that you're lying on your back with the right leg bent, foot flat on the floor close to the buttock. Place the left foot on the right thigh. Stretch the arms overhead and press the back and shoulders to the floor. In 4 slow counts, raise the arms up and forward as you elevate your head and shoulders. Aim the nose to your knee and bounce 4 times with the arms reaching forward. Lower to the floor. Change leg position (right foot on the left thigh) and repeat. Try this 6–8 times, alternating legs.

Advanced: Take the intermediate position. As you raise your head and shoulders on 4 counts, carry your arms out to the sides instead of bringing them forward. Bounce the nose to the knee for 6 counts, then return the head to the floor. Change legs and repeat. Practice 6–8 times, alternating legs.

Body Awareness: When you lift your head, pull the stomach in. Shoulders are relaxed, not hunched. This is a good exercise to strengthen the abdomen and to relieve low-back pain.

The Backpress

Position: Lie on your back, arms stretched overhead on the floor, legs together and toes pointed.

Beginners: Press your arms, shoulders, neck, and small of your back into the floor and hold for 8 counts. Release for 4. Repeat 6–8 times. As you press your back to the floor, shrink your stomach in and let the hips tilt up slightly.

Intermediates: Try the beginner version twice. On the third time, squeeze your buttocks very tightly together and lift your legs only a few inches off the floor. Hold for 4 counts, then relax for 4. Repeat 3 more times without letting the back arch off the floor.

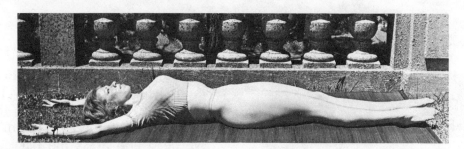

Advanced: Start with the beginner version, then try the intermediate version. Do each twice. The fifth time, tighten your buttocks and simultaneously lift your arms and legs a few inches off the floor. Stretching the arms long overhead and lengthening the legs in the opposite direction, hold for 6 counts. Relax for 4. Repeat 3 times.

Body Awareness: To avoid back strain, keep the small of the back and the shoulders pressed to the floor. If your back comes off the floor when the legs lift a few inches, then bring your legs up higher. Feel your spine stretching as the stomach and buttock muscles are being toned?

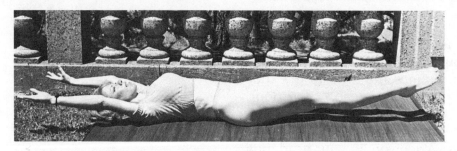

The Snail

If you suffer from stiff and achy back muscles, this exercise I call the Snail will bring relief and a gentle stretch.

Position: Get down on all fours. Flatten your back so that it is parallel to the floor, and draw your stomach in. Keep your head level.

Beginners: In 4 counts, slowly lower your seat to your heels and your chest to your thighs (or as close together as they can be). Place your arms behind you alongside the legs, hands next to feet, and hold the position for 8–12 counts. Return to the kneeling position in 4 counts. Repeat twice more, or as often as you like.

Wallhanging

This posture-correction exercise will gently stretch your back muscles, and will help prevent mild back pain.

Position: Stand with your arms, head, shoulders, and buttocks flush up against a wall.

Beginners: Place your heels about 4 inches from the wall and bend your knees slightly. Try to melt your lower back into the wall by shrinking and flattening the stomach. Tilt your hips (pelvis) up and tuck your buttocks under as you flatten the upper and lower back to the wall. Hold the position for 8 counts. Now slowly straighten your knees on 8 without letting your back lose wall-contact. Repeat the exercise 8–16 times, constantly melting the upper and lower back into the wall.

Intermediates and Advanced: Follow the beginner exercise, except with arms stretched overhead. Place the heels and arms against the wall, knees bent. Now slowly straighten your knees while keeping all parts in close contact with the wall (see photo).

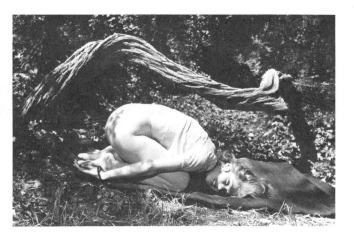

Intermediate and Advanced: As you lower your bottom to your heels, stretch the right arm forward on the floor and place the right ear on the floor. The left arm is behind you next to your legs. Hold the position for 4–6 slow counts, then change arms and ears for 4. Return to your hands and knees, then repeat twice or more.

Now stretch both your arms straight forward on the floor when you lower your bottom to your heels. Try to touch your forearms, elbows, and one ear on the floor as you hold for 8–12 counts. Return to all fours and repeat a couple of times or more if desired.

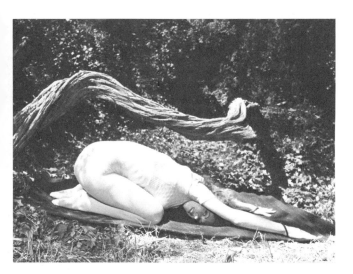

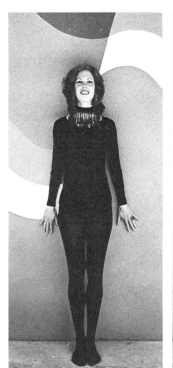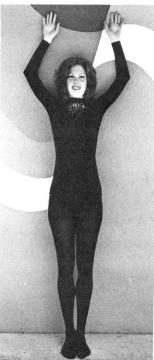

Body Awareness: Remember to retract your stomach throughout the exercise. Are you feeling the lower back muscles gently extending? In the advanced stage you should be feeling the shoulders and upper back muscles stretching.

Body Awareness: To keep your back flat, you'll need to draw the stomach muscles in tightly. Feel the back muscles stretching? This is an especially good exercise for those who suffer from low-back pain, and for those with a swayback or with rounded shoulders.

Caterpillar Crawl

(Crawling the Walls)

Nothing will burden your muscles or undo all the physical benefits gained from exercising more than a slumped, misaligned posture. Most of us pay little attention to the way we hold ourselves as we go about our daily routines. Consequently, we aren't aware of when we are burdening or benefiting our bodies. *All* movement is exercise, and if some basic posture principles are applied to everyday living, you won't ever have to feel as if you're dragging your body around with you. Concentrate on some simple ways to help improve your posture, beginning with this wall-crawling exercise.

Position: Lean up against a wall with your feet placed a few inches from it. Now drop forward and let yourself go limp as if you were hanging over a clothesline. Draw your stomach in.

Start: Slowly crawl your spine up the wall by pressing each vertebra, one by one, into the support. Concentrate first on pressing the lower back, then the upper back, shoulders, neck, and back of the head against the wall. When you've straightened up completely, hold the pressed position for several seconds. Bend over and repeat the exercise a second time. AFter you hold the flat-back position against the wall for a few seconds, step away and remember the feeling of extreme straightness. Try to hold the position on your own, then step back against the wall and check yourself. Practice this exercise as many times as you like during the day.

Body Awareness: You'll need to suck your stomach in deeply to keep your back flat against the wall. Some degree of curvature in the lower back is normal, but if your curve is exaggerated you will have difficulty flattening your lower back (if so, bend your knees slightly).

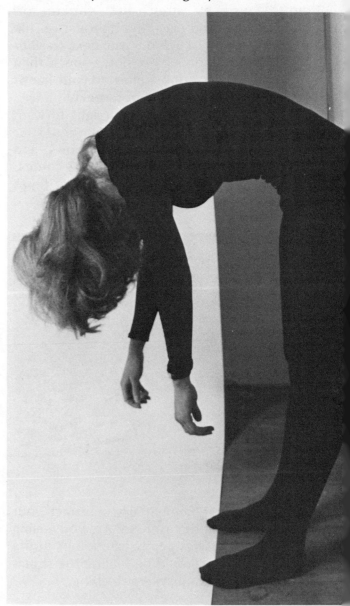

Flamingo

Since balance is such an important aspect to the success of most physical activities, it wouldn't hurt (literally) to practice staying on balance while you exercise. Here you'll also be giving your back and thighs a gentle stretch.

Position: Stand with your stomach drawn in and your spine lengthened. The left arm extends to the side and touches a wall or support. Lift one knee as close to your chest as possible and grasp it with the right hand. Think tall.

Beginners: Pull your knee up to your chest 8 times with toes pointed. Change knees and repeat. Now turn around so the right hand braces the wall, and repeat the set with the left hand pulling one knee, then the other, for 8 counts. Repeat the above set a second time. For the third set, bounce the knee to your chest 4 times with one hand on the wall, then 4 times without touching the wall. Change knees. Change sides and repeat.

Intermediates: Lift one knee up to your chest and clasp it with both hands. Bounce it up 8 times, then change knees for 8. Now brace the wall with one hand. Lift and grasp one knee to your chest as you raise up onto the ball of the standing foot. Hold up for 4 counts, then release your support and hug the knee with both hands as you balance-hold for 4 counts. About-face and repeat on the other side. Try the entire set once more each side.

Advanced: Brace a wall with the left hand and raise the left heel high off the floor. Raise the right knee to your chest and grasp it with the right hand. Now bounce the knee up to your chest 8 times while your left heel is raised. Release your support and hug the knee with both hands. Without lowering your heel, hold knee to chest for 8 counts. About-face and repeat the set. Practice the sets a second time.

Body Awareness: You can improve your balance if you concentrate on drawing your stomach in under you and lengthening your back and neck. Keep the standing leg very straight and strong (no wobbly knees). When you raise your knee, don't let the hip lift up with it. Keep both hips centered. Do you feel the thigh muscles stretching? You should also feel the feet and calves strengthening in the intermediate and advanced versions.

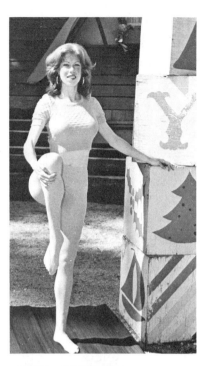

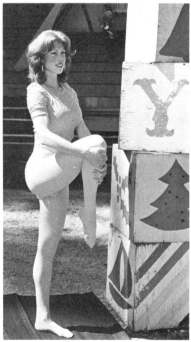

Spiral Stretch

The following three exercises are more demanding back stretches. This stretch will restore resiliency to stiff back muscles.

Position: Sit with your legs together, knees straight and toes pointed down. Flatten your stomach.

Beginners: Place your hands beside your knees. Draw the stomach in as you drop your chin to your chest. Slowly and gently bounce your head toward the knees 8 times, concentrating on rounding and closing your upper body as if you were spiraling into yourself. In 4 counts, straighten up to the starting position. Continue the exercise without pausing 4 or more times.

Intermediates: Lace your fingers behind your neck and point the elbows down. Follow the beginner exercise. As you spiral and bounce, try to touch your head to the knees but don't let the shoulders hunch up while bouncing. Repeat 8–12 (or more) times.

Advanced: Grasp your ankles, then round and close your upper body. Let the forehead touch the knees on each bounce. Repeat 8–16 (or more) times.

Body Awareness: Expect to feel a stretch in your back, especially in the middle back. Some students also feel a stretch along the backs of the thighs (hamstring muscles). Be sure your bounces are gentle, short, and smooth. You're cheating if your knees bend or your shoulders hunch up to your neck. Keep them down and relaxed. Try to shrink in the stomach throughout the exercise.

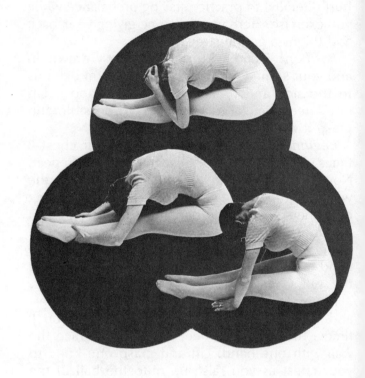

Pretzel Reach

Here's a three-way stretch for your back, buttocks, and chest. One of the most challenging aspects of this exercise is getting yourself into the position.

Position: Sit with your right leg folded, with the heel under your left buttock. Now cross the left leg over the right and place your left foot flat on the floor next to your right knee (keep your left knee pointed skyward). Slide the right knee forward slightly to tighten your leg position.

Beginners: 1. Straighten one arm overhead past your ear and, with a very straight back, pulsate your chest toward your right knee 12 times. Let the arm bounce back behind your ear when your chest pulsates forward. Change arms and repeat.

2. Now place both hands on the floor at your left side. Round over and bounce for 12 beats, aiming the top of your head as close to the floor as possible. Don't let the buttock and heel lose contact with each other. Repeat the set once or twice again.

Now that you've managed to get yourself into this position, try unwinding, then reversing it. Repeat the exercise 3 times on the second side.

Intermediates: Follow the beginner instructions carefully. In part 1, raise *both* arms overhead as you pulsate your chest to the knee.

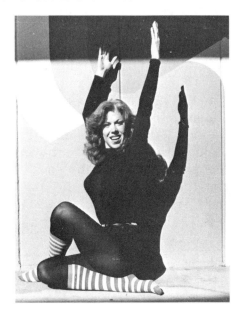

Advanced: Mimic the intermediate exercise. In part 2, when you round over you should be able to touch your head on the floor.

Body Awareness: You're cheating if you let your buttocks and heel separate from each other during any part of the exercise. In part 1 you should be feeling your back and chest stretching. In part 2, are you feeling a buttock and upper-thigh stretch?

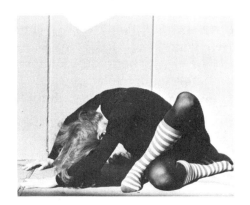

The Plow

The plow is one way to iron the kinks out of a stiff back.

Position: Lie on your back with your knees bent up to your chest. Place your arms at your sides with palms down.

Beginners: Straighten both legs up to the ceiling, keeping your toes pointed. As slowly as possible, push your hands against the floor while you lift your hips up. At the same time, thrust your legs overhead so your knees are above your forehead. If you start to roll down, prop your hips up by placing your hands at your lower back. Keep your knees straight and the legs together as you hold the position for 12–16 counts.

Now slowly lower your back and legs to the floor by rolling down your spine. Let your knees bend on the way down. Repeat the exercise 4–8 times.

Intermediates: Follow the beginner exercise and continue to stretch your legs overhead until your toes touch on the floor behind your head. Keep your arms on the floor (they don't prop your hips up in this case). Hold for 12 or more counts before rolling down your spine. Try to keep your legs straight on the way down. Perform 4–8 times.

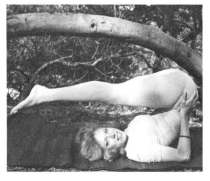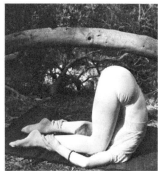

Advanced: Start with the intermediate version. After your toes touch the floor overhead, bend both knees alongside your ears on the floor. Hold the position for 12 or more counts, then straighten the legs overhead again. Slowly roll down your spine until your legs reach the floor. Repeat four times.

Body Awareness: Keep your chin tucked in and pressing on your chest. This exercise may appear frightening to accomplish, but really, it looks harder than it actually is. Perform it in gradual steps and you'll adjust to the topsy-turvy feeling of having your legs overhead. Are you feeling a stretch from the lower back all the way up to your neck?

Bedtime Back Exercise

Position: Lie on your back with your lower legs propped on the bed (or chair) and your hips flush up against the edge, at a 90-degree angle to the floor. Lie in this position for a minute. Feel your spine, shoulders, and neck melting into the floor while you try to suck your stomach in. Try to hold this position for several seconds (keep breathing naturally).

Start: Raise one leg skyward. Point the toes and strive to straighten your knee. If the muscles behind your thigh are tight, then you won't be able to straighten the leg completely.

Pulsate the leg toward your chest (without hold-ing it) for 16 slow beats. Be sure that you don't let the shoulders lift off the floor or the knee bend any more than when you started.

Now grasp your calf with both hands and try to touch your head to your knee. Hold the position for 4–8 counts, then return to starting position. Change legs and repeat the sequence. Repeat the exercise once or twice more.

Body Awareness: Remember to keep your stomach in throughout the exercise. Expect to feel a stretch along the back of the legs and in the lower back. Try this back exercise twice daily—upon awakening and retiring.

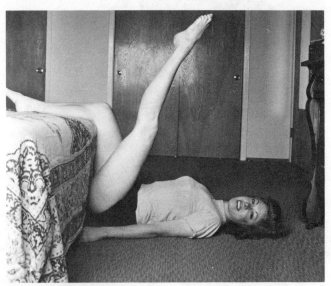

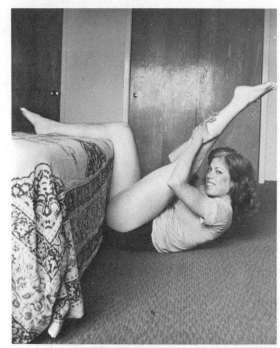

The Technique: Back-Hamstring Connection (Challenging Stretches for Normal Backs)

Warm-up Bounces I

One way to prevent low-back strain is to keep the long back and hamstring muscles very limber. This exercise helps you attain maximum flexibility while it relaxes your entire body.

Position: Stand with feet wide apart, toes parallel and knees straight.

Beginners: Place hands on hips and bend over to the right leg from the buttocks, not from the waist. Your back should be parallel with the floor. As you bend, be sure the back is flat (no rounded shoulders). Keep your head up, shoulder blades drawn together, elbows up, and stomach pulled

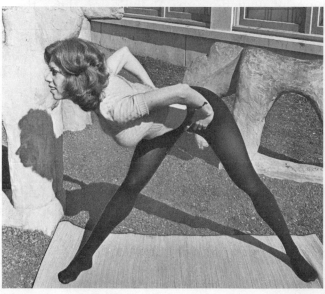

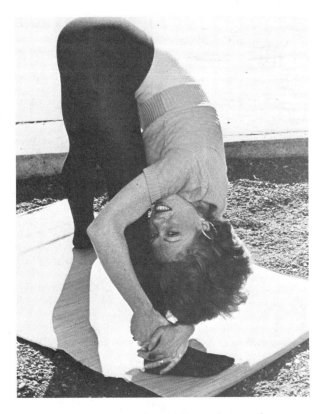

in. When you've lowered halfway down, bounce slowly and gently toward the right leg for 10 counts. Straighten up and repeat to the left side. Continue the set 3–4 more times, alternating sides.

Try to pulsate a little closer to the leg with each bounce. Are you feeling the muscle down the back of each leg stretch as you bounce?

Intermediates: Start with the beginner version. For the next 3–4 sets, grasp your calf and gently pull into the leg as you bounce. You cheat if you bend a knee or if the shoulders round.

Advanced: Bending with a flat back, grasp your right ankle with both hands. Slowly lower your chest onto the right thigh, and let your left ear touch your right kneecap! Gently pulsate down for 8 beats before changing sides. Repeat 3–6 times per leg.

Body Awareness: You can flatten your back by drawing the stomach muscles in constantly. As you gently bounce, aim the upper torso closer to the leg without letting the shoulders droop. This exercise also serves as a good warm-up stretch to precede any sport endeavor.

Contrary to popular belief, gentle, rhythmic bouncing while you stretch is a very effective and safe way to improve your flexibility. Dancers in particular have used this "ballistic" method for decades with great success. Just remember to position yourself correctly (follow the instructions) and keep your bounces gentle rather than vigorous.

Warm-up Bounces II

> **CAUTION;** *The back-arch is not for people with low-back problems.*

Position: Stand with feet wide apart, toes parallel, and knees pulled straight.

Beginners: Place hands on hips. Bend forward, slowly, with a flat back. Keep the head up, shoulder blades drawn together, and stomach pulled in. Feel the muscles behind both legs stretching! When you have bent forward (from the buttocks, not from the waist) to your stretch limit, bounce gently 8–12 times. Come up and begin to arch back. Let your head drop back. Bounce with an arched back 8–12 times. Repeat the set 3–4 more times, alternating forward and back.

Intermediates: Start with the beginner version. For the next 3–4 sets, grasp both calves when you bend forward. With each bounce, pull your upper body toward the space between the legs. Straighten up, then arch way back and bounce back with hands on hips and shoulder blades drawn together. Repeat 3–4 times.

Advanced: Bend forward with a flat back and grasp both ankles. Bounce 8–12 times by pulling into the legs, head between the knees. Take 4 counts to straighten up, then arch way back. With hands on the back of your knees, pulsate back 8 times, trying to see the floor behind you. Come up and repeat the set 3–4 times.

Body Awareness: When arching back, don't tense the shoulders. Keep the shoulder tips pressed down. If you let your knees bend, then you'll lose the stretch benefits.

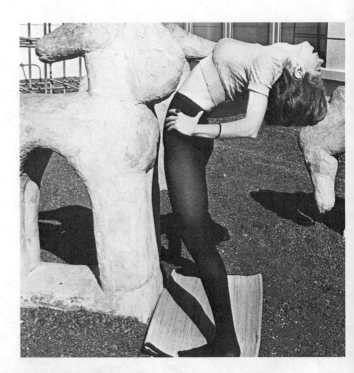

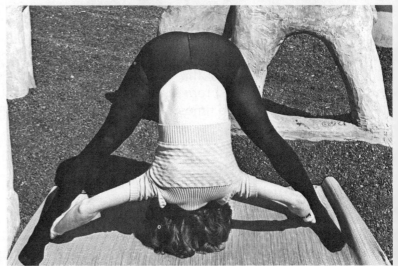

The Ostrich

The Ostrich is a good leg-and-back stretch, but should be preceded by simple warm-up stretches, such as warm-up bounces.

Position: Stand with legs as far apart as possible, so that the inner thigh muscles feel a stretch but aren't being pulled painfully. (Be careful!) Feet should be parallel.

Beginners: Try to touch hands to the floor, bending slowly from the hips with a flat, straight back. Bend the knees to let palms touch the floor. Drop your head down and bounce 8 times. Try to get your head closer to the floor with each bounce.

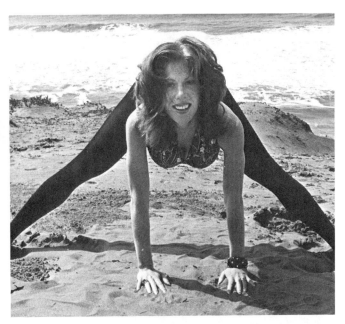

From this position, stretch the arms straight out past the ears, parallel to the floor, and straighten your legs. Hold with a nice, flat back for 4 counts. Return your hands to the floor and repeat the sequence at least twice.

Intermediates: The knees should be straight as you touch the top of your head to the floor.

Advanced: Legs should be wide apart. As your forehead and elbows reach the floor, try to feel as though you are burrowing into it like an ostrich. Hold for 8 counts, then stretch arms out as above.

Body Awareness: Pulling the stomach in helps to elongate and flatten the back. To avoid neck and shoulder tension, keep pressing your shoulder tips down and back. Can you feel your back and leg muscles stretching?

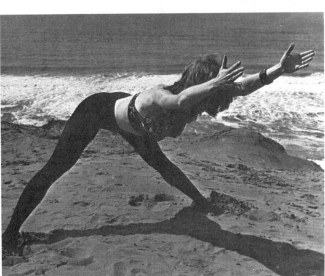

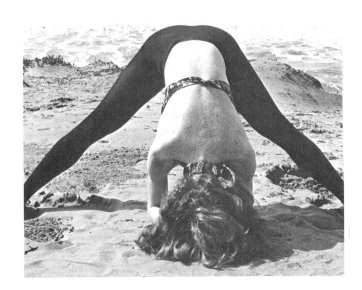

The Bouncer

This "bouncer" is a full stretch that increases suppleness in the back of the legs and back muscles.

Position: Squat all the way down with feet together, heels raised, and hands flat on the floor. Your chest should be touching your thighs.

Beginners: Bounce your bottom to your heels in the above position 8 times. Then half-straighten the knees and arms (4 counts). With your head and chest touching your legs, hold the half-straight position for 4 counts. Repeat the set 4–8 times without pausing.

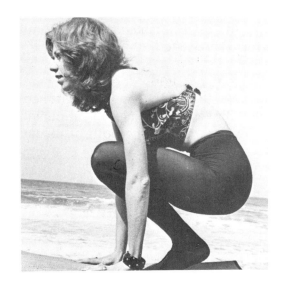

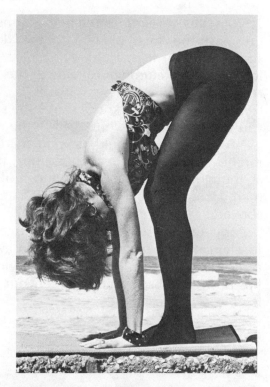

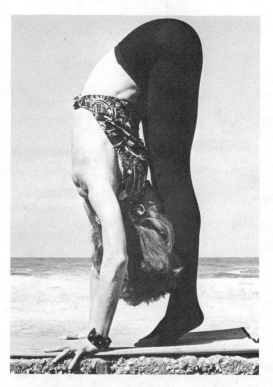

Intermediates: After bouncing for 8, keep the palms flat on the floor as you straighten your knees and elbows. Try to keep the upper torso as close to your legs as you can, but do heed signals from your muscles warning you of their stretch limit! Repeat the set 4–8 times without pausing.

Advanced: As you completely straighten the legs from the bounce, keep your heels raised. Hold straight for 4 before bouncing down again. Try the set 4–6 times.

Body Awareness: Press the shoulder tips down as you straighten your legs to avoid strain in the shoulders and upper back. Pulling the stomach in helps lengthen the long back muscles. You're cheating if your palms come off the floor!

Lunge-Stretch

Here's a super leg-and-thigh stretch that loosens the heel cord, the calves, hamstrings, and inner thighs. Use this exercise to limber up before any sport.

Position: Lunge the right foot forward and bend the right knee over the toes. Keep your right heel flat on the floor. Stretch the left leg straight behind you and lift the heel. Now place both hands flat at your sides.

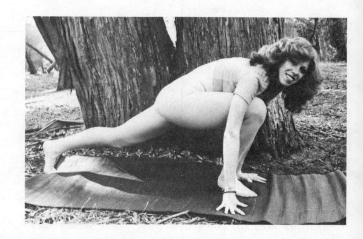

Beginners: Bounce up and down gently 8 times in the above lunge position (feel the inner thighs stretching?). Now *slowly* try to raise up by straightening the right leg as much as possible. Keep your hands flat on the floor and don't let your back knee bend. Hold this stretch position for 8–12 counts, then return to the lunge position. Don't expect to be able to straighten your front leg completely. Repeat both parts of the exercise, lunge-bounce and straighten-hold, for 4 sets in succession before changing legs. Pause, then repeat the entire sequence.

Intermediates: Follow the beginners' exercise, except straighten your front knee completely after the lunge. Now try to touch your chest to your thigh while you hold the standing position for 8–12 counts.

Advanced: Gently bounce 8 times in the lunge position, then straighten the front knee completely and raise the toes off the floor. Now touch your chest to your front thigh and your ear to your knee. Hold it there for 8–12 slow counts. Return to the lunge position and repeat the exercise 4

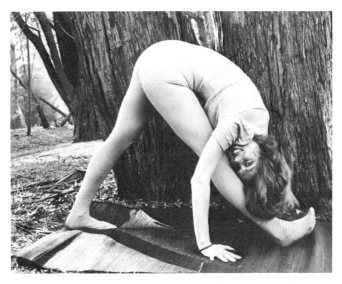

times. Switch leg positions and continue for another 4 sets. Repeat the sequence.

Body Awareness: Beginning students want to bend the back knee, but by doing so, much of the stretch benefit is lost. Try to keep the back leg very straight to restore maximum elasticity to the leg muscles.

Lunge-Kick

Here's an exercise that develops a multitude of muscles. You'll be toning and contouring the thighs, strengthening the stomach, and stretching the calves, the lower back, and the hamstrings.

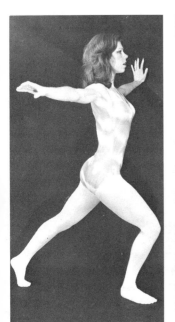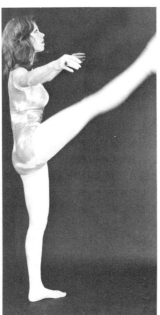

Position: Assume a lunge position with the right foot forward, knee bent over the toes. Stretch the left leg way behind the right and straighten the left knee. Touch one hand to a wall for support, stretch the other arm sideways, and draw your stomach in. Now think tall.

Beginners: Thump your back heel up and down on the floor for 3 counts. On the 4th count, swing-kick the back leg forward and up to waist height. As you energetically kick the leg, point your toes and straighten both knees. Be sure you're not rounding your back or shoulders. Immediately return to the lunge position and repeat the 3 thumps and 1 high kick. Continue for 8 sets on one side. Immediately about-face and repeat on the other side for 8 sets. Relax, then repeat the sequence once or twice more.

Intermediates: Stretch your arms to the sides and, without touching a wall for support, follow the beginner exercise. You should be able to kick your leg a little higher than waist level. Remember that bending the knees when you kick is subtly cheating.

Advanced: Each kick should thrust your leg up to the same height as your head. Perform the exercise without touching the wall for support.

Body Awareness: At the very same moment that you kick, pull your stomach in. You're cheating if you let your shoulders or back round. Keep thinking tall! Are you enjoying all of the stretching and strengthening you feel in your legs and back?

Wishbone

This balance exercise stretches the back and thighs while it strengthens the front thighs and stomach.

Position: Sit with knees bent and open to the sides. Feet are together and close to the body. Straighten your back.

Beginners: Grasp the right heel from the inside with your right hand. Slowly try to straighten the right leg up and out to the right side. Carry the leg only as high and as straight as you can without letting your back get round. Hold the leg up for 6 counts, trying to lengthen the back and leg. Take it down and change sides. Repeat at least 4 times on each side.

Intermediates: Start with the beginner exercise. When the right leg is straightened out to the side, hold it as you carry the left leg up and out. Balance on your buttocks, forming a wishbone with your legs. Hold for 4 counts, then bring the legs down. Repeat at least twice more.

Advanced: Straighten both legs up and out simultaneously. When you feel balanced, let go of the heels and hold the legs up for 8 counts without letting them drop in height. Repeat twice more.

Body Awareness: If you let your back get round, you will lose your balance and roll backward. Pulling the stomach in and lifting the chest will help flatten your back. Feel muscles along the inner thighs, back of the legs, and in the back stretching?

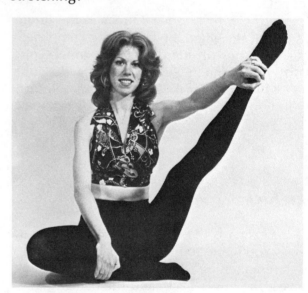

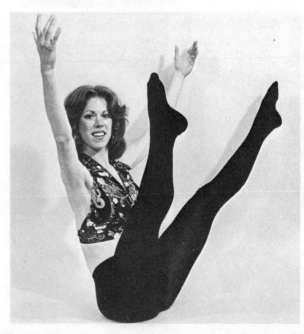

Lying Bent-Knee Pulls

Try this back-and-thigh stretch next time tension and muscular rigidity set in.

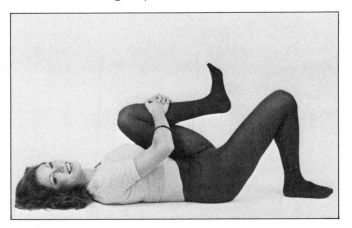

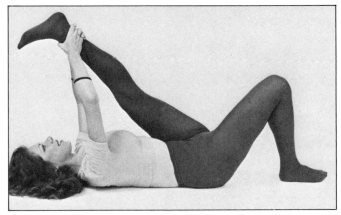

Position: Lie on your back with knees bent and feet flat on the floor, close to your buttocks. Shrink in your stomach.

Beginners: Hug one knee close to your chest and bounce it to you 8 times with foot flexed up. Now try to straighten the leg skyward, toes pointed. Stop when you feel a pull behind the knee (don't expect the leg to completely straighten). Now grasp the leg from behind the thigh with both hands and gently pulsate it closer to your chest for 8 slow counts. Repeat for 8 with the toes pointed. Now draw the leg as close to you as possible without lifting your hips or shoulders off the floor, and hold for 8 more counts. (Your knee is still bent.) Change legs and repeat. Try the entire exercise at least once or twice more.

Intermediates: Follow the beginner exercise except with your raised leg kept very straight. Grasp your knee or calf when you pulsate the leg toward you.

Advanced: Perform the beginner exercise with the raised leg kept very straight, and with both hands grasping the ankle.

Body Awareness: You're cheating if you let one hip lift up, or if you raise your head and shoulders off the floor. Are you feeling the muscles all along the back of your leg stretching? You might also feel a stretch in your lower back.

Lying Leg Pulls

This exercise, which helps to relieve or prevent low-back pain and stiff legs, is more difficult than the preceding one.

Position: Lie on your back with the knees bent and feet flat on the floor. Shrink your stomach so you feel as though your back (and shoulders) are melting into the floor.

Beginners: 1. Hug one knee to your chest and bounce it to you 8 times while you point the toes.

2. Now try to straighten the leg to the ceiling. Stop when you feel a pull behind the knee (don't expect the leg to straighten completely). Grasp the leg from behind the knee with both hands and gently pulsate it closer to your chest for 8 slow counts.

3. Now draw the leg as close to you as possible and hold for 8 counts with the toes pointed (your knee is still bent).

Hug the knee to your chest again and repeat the entire exercise set with the same leg. This time, instead of pointing the toes, flex them back by pushing through your heel when you straighten the leg. Change legs for 2 sets (once with toes pointed; once with them flexed). Repeat the sets twice with each leg for 4–8 rounds.

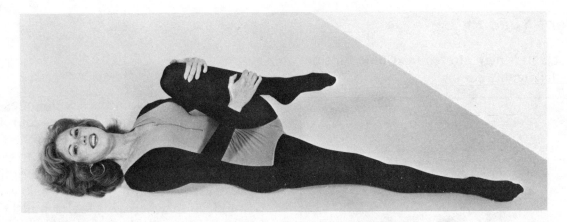

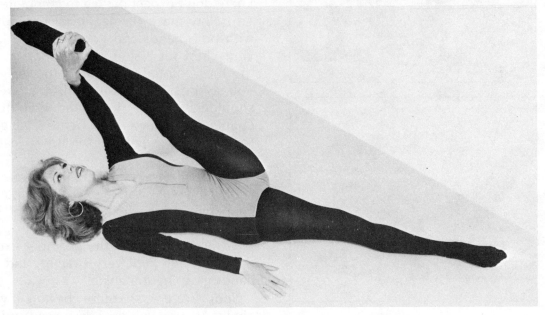

Intermediates: Follow the beginner exercise. Your leg should be completely straight in steps 2 and 3.

Advanced: In steps 2 and 3, grasp your right ankle with your right hand when you completely straighten and bounce the leg toward you. Change legs and hands for 6–8 rounds.

Body Awareness: Expect to feel the muscles stretch in your lower back and along the back of your thighs to the knee. Be sure not to let your lower back arch off the floor. You're cheating if you raise your shoulders or hips off the floor.

Banana Splits

A luxurious stretch to gain more flexible, supple inner-thigh, hamstring, and back muscles.

Position: Sit with your legs stretched as far apart as possible. Point the toes and flatten the knees to the floor. Place your hands on the floor behind you close to the buttocks. As you press your hands into the floor, lengthen and straighten your back.

Beginners: Sit with your back against a support if the above position is uncomfortable in the lower back region. Grasp your right knee with both hands and face the leg. In 4 slow counts, bend from your hips halfway down to the leg. Hold the position for 8 beats. Keep the back flat as you lean (no rounded shoulders). Now bounce toward the leg gently and slowly (take it easy) for 8 counts. Keep your head up. Hold for 8 counts, then bounce down again for 8. Repeat 3 times to one leg, then 3 sets to the other leg. Repeat the sequence a second time.

Intermediates: Follow the beginner version, grasping the ankle instead of the knee. As you bounce and hold, your chest should be closer to your thigh.

Advanced: Grasp the heel with both hands. Lower your chest to the thigh. As you bounce very gently and slowly, feel your inner-thigh and waist muscles stretch. When you hold for 8, try to touch your ear to the knee.

Body Awareness: You're cheating if your shoulders round, if one buttock lifts off the floor, or if you let a knee bend and rotate forward (keep the knees facing up at the ceiling). My students discover the luxurious feeling from the total stretch this exercise gives, from the pointed toes up through the legs, waistline, back, and out through the arms.

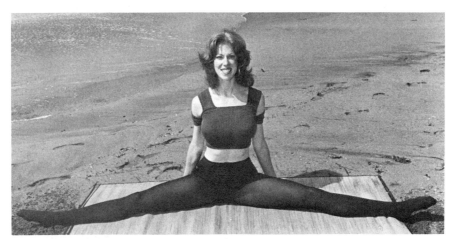

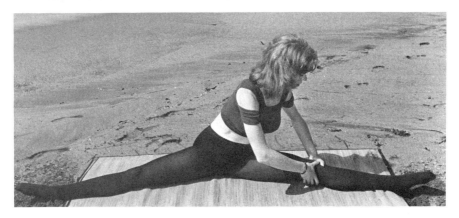

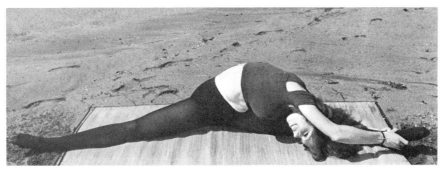

Sideways Splits

A luxurious stretch that helps trim the waist and restore elasticity to the inner-thigh and hamstring muscles.

Position: Sit with legs as wide apart as possible so your muscles feel stretched, but not overpulled. Point your toes and straighten your knees. Straighten your spine.

Beginners: You may want to sit with your back and hips against a wall for support. Grasp your right knee and arc your left arm overhead. Stretch sideways to your right leg as you bounce—gently and slowly—to the right for 8 counts. Do you feel a luxurious stretch extending up your left side as you bounce? Now hold the sideways stretch for 8 counts.

Change arms and stretch-bounce and hold to the left for 8 counts. Repeat the set once or twice more in each direction before bringing the legs together and shaking them out.

Intermediates: Follow the beginner exercise but hold your legs farther apart. As you gently bounce sideways, strive to lower your waist closer to your leg.

Advanced: Place your right elbow and forearm on the floor alongside the inner part of your right leg. Grasp underneath your right ankle with your right hand. Lengthen your left arm overhead, close to your left ear, as you bounce sideways 8 times, and then hold close to your leg for 8 counts. Now just reach the overhead arm way back behind you and twist your upper torso up and back, striving to open your chest to the ceiling. Feel a superstretch along your midriff! Repeat the entire set once or twice more on each side.

Body Awareness: You're cheating if you let one buttock lift off the floor, if you bend a knee or elbow, or if you let your knees turn forward (keep them facing the ceiling). I warn beginners not to attempt the wide sitting position until the inner-thigh muscles have developed enough elasticity.

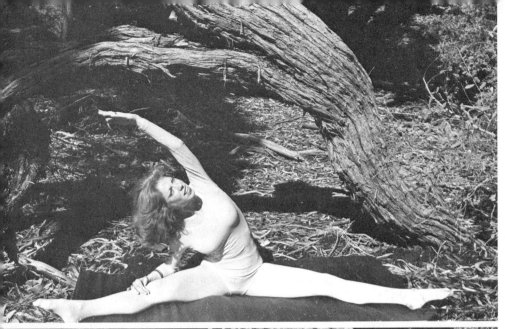

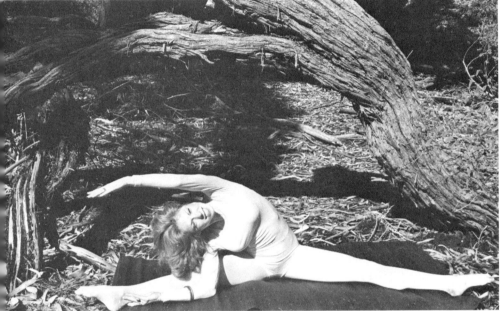

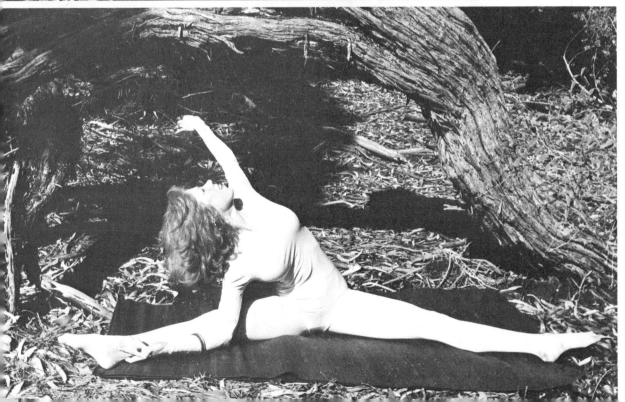

Forward Splits

With gradual and consistent practice, this exercise will free a stiff back and inner thighs.

Position: Sit on the floor with your feet flexed up and your legs spread as wide apart as possible so you feel an inner-thigh stretch (be careful not to overstrain). Straighten your spine and draw your stomach in.

Beginners: If you find it difficult to keep your back straight in this position, then sit with your hips and back flush up against a wall. Place your hands on the floor in front of you and, keeping your back very flat, lean over as far forward as you can.

Gently bounce forward for 8 slow counts, striving to aim your chest closer to the floor with each bounce. Hold for 8, then bounce for 8 more. Continue alternating the 8-count bounce-hold for 4 sets. Straighten up, bring the legs together and shake them out, then repeat the sequence. Perform the exercise a third time.

Intermediates: Follow the beginner instructions with your legs further apart. You should be able to keep your hands and forearms on the floor throughout the exercise.

Advanced: Split your legs wide apart. You won't be able to stretch them out to 180 degrees, but you *might* be able to come close! Slowly and gently pulsate forward and strive to touch your upper torso and arms to the floor. Do be careful not to overpull the inner-thigh muscles! Now try to hold the position for 8–12 counts, then bring the legs together, shake them out, and repeat the exercise.

Body Awareness: You're cheating if you let your back round, your stomach pop out, or your knees bend. To keep the feet flexed, push through your heels. Are you feeling a superstretch along the inner thighs?

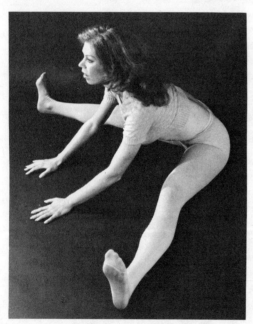
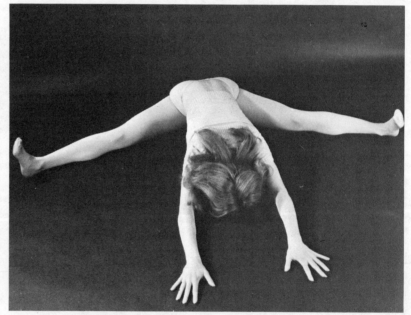

Long Stretch Forward

To help limber your waist, back, and thigh muscles, thereby avoiding that morning-after stiffness from sports or dancing.

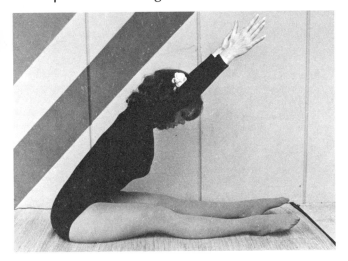
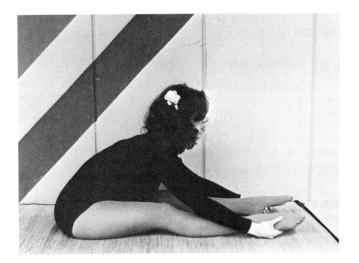
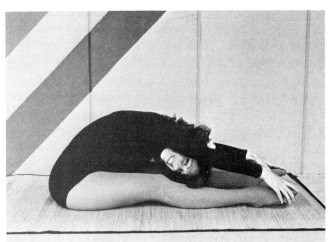

Position: Sit with your legs straight and toes pointed. Lengthen your back to its utmost and flatten the stomach. Press the tips of your shoulders down as you straighten your arms past your ears.

Beginners: You may sit against a wall if you feel strain in the lower back when it is unsupported. Keeping your back straight, reach forward. Bend from the hips to about halfway down. Bounce slowly and gently 10 times. Straighten up on 4 counts, then repeat for at least 3 more sets.

Intermediates: Follow the beginner instructions, only bend lower from the hips so that your chest is closer to your thighs and you can grasp your feet. Hold there for 8 counts, then bounce for 8. Repeat the hold-bounce set 3 times before straightening up. Relax, then repeat for another 3 sets.

Advanced: Bend all the way down so that your upper torso rests on your thighs and your ear touches the knees. Hold the position for 8 counts, then gently bounce for 8. Repeat the set twice more before straightening up. Try the set again.

Body Awareness: For maximum flexibility benefits, keep the back and knees very straight. Try not to let your arms drop below your ears when you gently bounce. You should feel muscles in the back, waist, and behind the knees really lengthening.

The Technique: Challenging Backward Stretches—for healthy backs only.

Small Bridges

This one stretches your back, strengthens your thighs, and tones your buttocks. It even helps relieve menstrual cramps!

Position: Lie on your back with your knees bent up and feet flat on the floor about shoulder-width apart. Rest your arms at your sides and draw your stomach in gently.

Beginners: Raise your hips 3 or 4 inches off the floor. Keeping them high, bounce your pelvis gently toward the sky for 12 counts without touching the floor. Now curl your back down on the floor from the shoulders to the base of your spine. Repeat 4 times.

Intermediates: Follow the beginner version but raise your hips as high off the floor as you can. Bounce the pelvis skyward for 16 counts before curling down. Repeat 4–6 times.

Advanced: Perform one set of the intermediate exercise. While your hips are still raised high, lift one leg skyward. Point your toes and straighten the knee as you hold your leg up for 8, then slowly curl your back down to the floor. Repeat 4 times.

Body Awareness: While bouncing your hips up, you can tone the back of your thighs and buttocks if you consciously squeeze them together. Are you also feeling the front thigh muscles building strength? If you are a ski buff, try this exercise daily before you head for snow.

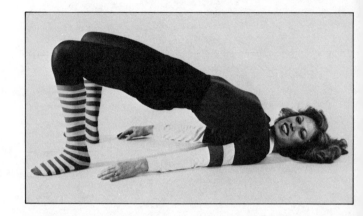

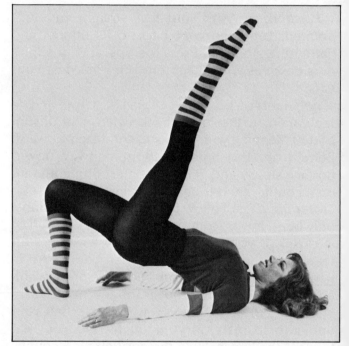

Back-Bend Bridge

While strengthening your back, this super exercise stretches the chest, arms, and abdominal muscles.

Position: Lie on your back with knees and elbows bent. Palms are flat on the floor next to your ears.

Beginners: Pressing down evenly with your hands and feet, raise only your hips, then back, as high as possible off the floor. Hold the lift for 4 counts, then return to the floor. Repeat 2 to 4 times.

Intermediates: Let your shoulders and neck lift up so the top of your head is on the floor. Your elbows will begin to straighten. Hold for 4, then lower to the floor. Repeat 2–4 times.

Advanced: Lift up so that only your hands and feet remain on the floor. Straighten the elbows. Try walking your hands and feet closer together so you deepen the back roll. Lower and repeat twice.

Body Awareness: You may find this upside-down position uncomfortable or even frightening at first. With gradual, consistent practice it will become easier to relax into the back bend so you can drop your head and deepen your arch. Do you feel your neck, back, and abdominal muscles stretching?

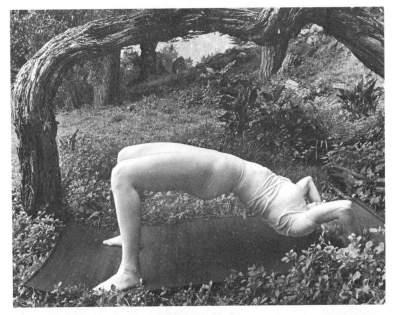

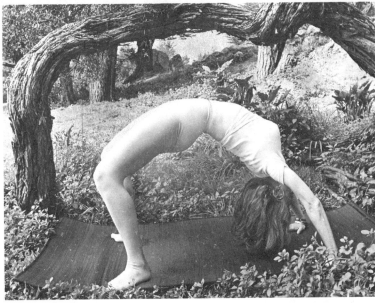

Off Your Rocker

Another complete body stretch.

Position: Lie on your stomach with legs apart and bent up. Hands are grasping the ankles. If you are on a bare floor, you may want to cushion the hip bones.

Beginners: Pull only the thighs as high off the floor as possible. Hold them up for 4 counts before lowering them to the floor. Repeat at least 3 more times. Feel the top thigh muscles stretching?

Intermediates: Lift the thighs and chest off the floor simultaneously. Arch way back and up. Hold 4 counts before relaxing. Repeat 3 more times, each time trying to lift and arch higher off the floor.

Advanced: When the chest and thighs are lifted to their maximum, rock forward and back on the hip bones 3 times. Relax, then repeat. Try not to drop the arch while rocking.

Body Awareness: Feel every muscle reaching upward, especially those in the back, neck, thighs, and stomach!

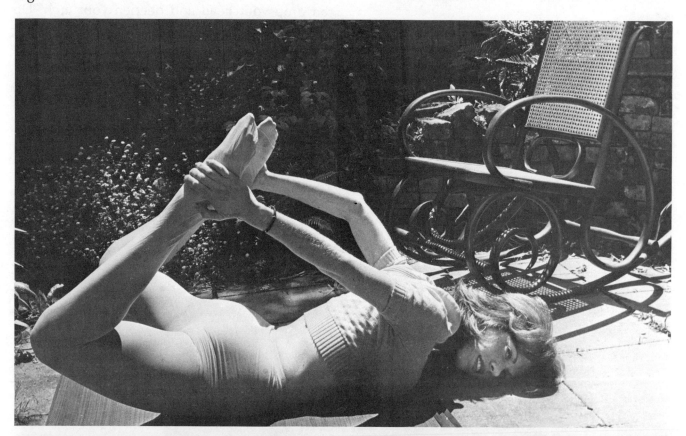

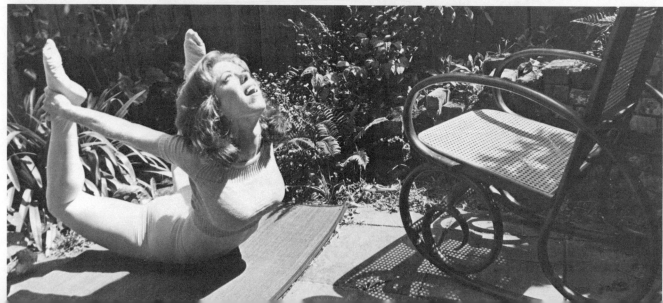

The Cobra

CAUTION: *Not for people with low-back problems.*

The Cobra will help those seeking a good back stretch.

Position: Lie on your stomach with hands at sides of chest, legs and feet touching.

Beginners: Squeezing buttocks together, raise your upper torso and try to straighten the elbows (4 counts to come up as high as possible). Hold up for 4 counts, then lower to the floor. Repeat 3 more times.

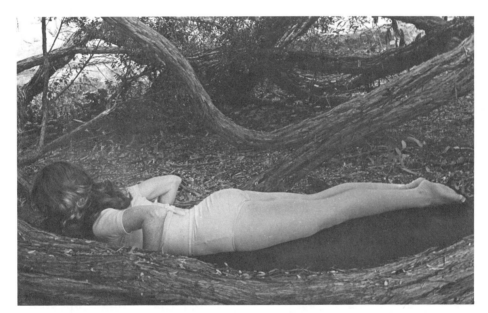

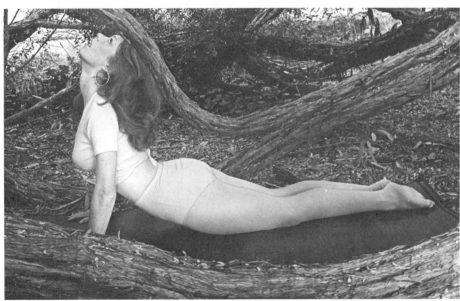

Intermediates and Advanced: While your upper torso is raised, drop your head and arch back as far as possible. Hold (4 counts). Lower and repeat 3 more times.

Body Awareness: Feet, legs and buttocks are all squeezing together. Feel the lower back, stomach, and neck muscles stretching as the buttock muscles are being toned.

The Pony

> CAUTION; *The intermediate and advanced versions may not be for you if you have a bad lower back.*

This Pony arching exercise will strengthen your abdomen and stretch your back simultaneously. The image of a pony will help to position you correctly for the exercise.

Position: Kneel on all fours with knees and feet a few inches apart. Flatten your back and level your head so you are smooth from head to tail.

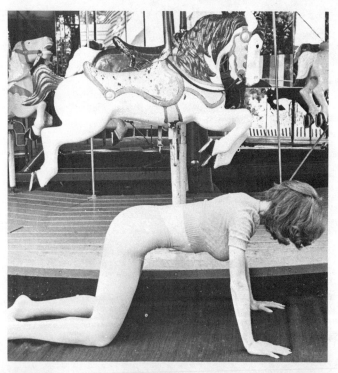

Beginners: Contract your stomach muscles, squeeze your buttocks together, and tuck in your hips in 4 counts. Then round and stretch your back up and let your head drop down in 4 counts. Hold this position for 4 counts as you press evenly on your hands and knees. Return to the beginning position in 4 counts. Repeat the exercise 6–10 times or as long as stamina permits. Remember to keep your stomach pulled in tightly.

Intermediates: Do the beginner version 3 times. The 4th time, instead of rounding your back and dropping your head, raise your chin high and drop your back into a sway. Hold this position for 4 counts, then return to a flat back. Repeat the set (round, flat, sway, flat) 6–8 times or as stamina permits.

Advanced: Round the back in 4 counts, release it, and dip it into a sway in 4, eliminating the flat-back position. Perform the set 4 times in 4 counts, then 4 times in 2 counts, then 4 times in 1 count. As you progress, the exercises should flow together without a pause.

Body Awareness: Just the stomach, back, and neck muscles should be working. If you hunch your shoulders, they will tense. Remember to keep your weight evenly distributed on your hands and knees. You're cheating if your elbows bend!

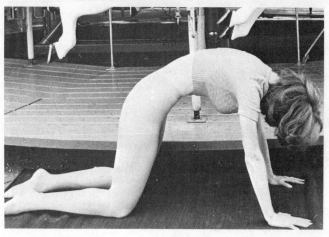

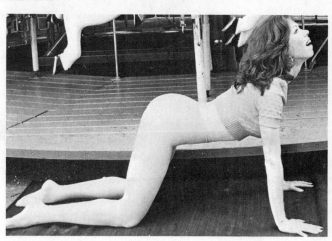

Unravel

The most effective way to unravel a tense body (and mind) is through exercise. Here is one simple movement that helps you release any pent-up tension.

Position: Sit on your heels and fold your torso over so that your chest is on your thighs and your head drops to your knees. Grasp your ankles and just relax for a few seconds in this curled-up position.

Start by slowly uncurling your way up until you arrive at a fully arched position. Use 5 slow counts to unravel into a full, high arch. Hold the arch for 3 counts as you let your head drop way back. Now contract the stomach muscles and fold down again in 5 counts by sitting on your heels first. Then curl over into the starting position. Repeat the exercise 6 times in succession so that you fold and unravel in one continuous motion.

Body Awareness: Don't let your arch collapse; you should be feeling more stretch in the front of your thighs. If your knees hurt during the exercise, cushion them or perform on a rug. Are you feeling your neck, shoulders, arms, chest, and thighs all stretching simultaneously?

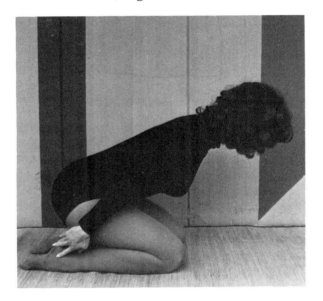
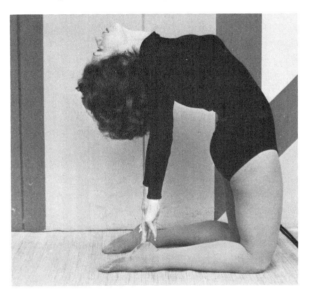

Backpainless Tips

● Standing in one place for long periods produces backaches, usually due to relaxing the stomach and buttock muscles allowing the lower back to sway. If possible, try to rest each foot alternately on a foot rail (or low footstool). By lifting your foot you straighten your lower back.
● If you have to stand for long periods, do it in shoes with low (one-inch) heels; it's easier on your back.
● Sleep on a firm bed, on your side (not your stomach), with knees bent up in a fetal position.
● Whenever you bend (whether the knees are straight or bent), always keep your back elongated. Even when you lean forward, lean from the hips with a straight spine.
● When lifting any heavy object, stand close to it, put one foot slightly ahead of the other, then bend the knees completely while keeping the back straight. Lift the object close to you with the same long back and flat stomach.
● To push or pull heavy objects, take a wide stance and bend the knees, but keep the back straight.
● When driving, sit close enough so your knees bend when they touch the pedals.
● The best sitting posture for low-back pain is with a pillow at the low back and the feet up, or knees bent up higher than the hips.
● If you climb stairs leaning too far forward, you're in for back strain. Keep erect or lean *slightly* forward.

CHAPTER FOUR:

HOW TO TONE AND TRIM YOUR THIGHS

Let's face it, gorgeous thighs are a true mark of aesthetic beauty. A pair of tapering, curvaceous, slim limbs gently molded from firm hips down to symmetrically positioned knees is a real work of art. Underlying every sculptured, contoured curve is a pair of shapely, long limbs are steel-strong muscles.

The thigh muscles are by far among the most powerful in your body. Extending from hip to knee, the thigh bones are the very largest, heaviest, and longest bones. They make up about one quarter of the entire length of your body. Your thighs can easily handle weights that can be too much of a strain for the arm and back muscles to maneuver. As the weight-bearers for your upper body, the thighs are your source of strength and stability when you stand or walk. Thighs serve to fortify the less-stable knees and hips by helping them to bend, straighten, and rotate.

The inner and outer thigh muscles are among the most neglected in the body. They were meant for continuous use, but a modern person's limited locomotive movements offer little need to engage their assistance daily, except for bending. They deteriorate from disuse and, especially in women, form ugly little fatty pads above the knees and just below the hips. The flab may appear dimpled like the peel of an orange skin or lumpy like cottage cheese. Weak inner and outer thigh muscles can instigate misalignments such as knock-knees or bowlegs, which need correction by strengthening the thigh muscles.

Men typically spend considerable time at building strength in their front thigh muscles to the neglect of restoring elasticity to the hamstrings, and to stiff inner, outer, and front thigh muscles. Women tend to be more supple in these areas, but need to strengthen and tone limp or fatty limbs. Through dieting and directly exercising them daily, the flaccid flesh can be effectively attacked. By the way, the very same exercises that contour and streamline thick thighs will also help to build up skinny ones.

I've divided the thigh exercises into two kinds. Most of this chapter consists of exercises to contour and tone loose muscles. Once you master the thigh-strengthening exercises in the advanced stages, you may want to add ankle weights or even a barbell for more development in less time. The last 6 exercises give you specific front and inner-thigh stretches.

Whenever you bend over and feel an arresting pull behind your thighs, you're awakening your hamstring muscles. The hamstrings are in the back of your thighs, extending from your sitting bones down to the bend in your knees. They help to flex the knees, extend the hips, and rotate your thighs together. If the hamstrings aren't kept resilient, they become as unyielding as barbed wire! Fossilized hamstrings give you an annoying pull down the back of your thighs when you dare to just casually bend over. Like tight reins yanking an old horse, they also prevent your back from stretching and straightening out completely when you try to sit up straight or lie down flat. In the chapter on back exercises, the section "Back-Hamstring Connection," you will find all the hamstring-stretching exercises you will ever need in life!

Whatever your goal, the rewards for your efforts will be rapidly realized because—cheer up—the thigh muscles respond to strengthening and stretching exercises more quickly than do most other body parts. As the thighs awaken to their full power and pliancy, your movements from the hips down will become liberated and, rather than dragging your body through life, they will enliven it for you!

Strengthening Technique

Diamond Knee Bends

Usually due to heredity, women will have a tendency to deposit excess fat around the buttocks and thighs. To develop any muscle tone in these areas takes a concerted effort, doing several kinds of exercises. This thigh-toner is one way to strengthen and contour floppy thigh muscles.

Beginners: Stand with heels about 2 feet apart and toes turned out slightly so they face east and west. Draw your stomach in, elongate your back, and place hands on hips. In 4 slow counts, bend knees as low as possible over the toes without lifting your heels off the floor. Don't let the knees fall forward, keep them wide open over the toes. Hold for 8 counts, then straighten up on 4 slow counts by squeezing your buttocks and inner thighs together. Repeat 6–8 times, each time drawing the inner thighs together as you straighten your knees.

Intermediates: Place the heels together, then follow the beginner exercise. As you open and bend your knees over the toes, try to form a wide diamond of space between the legs. Strive to bend as low as you can with your heels glued to the floor.

Advanced: Follow the intermediate version by bending the knees in two counts. Now continue bending all the way down as you lift your heels and keep them together. When you bend, your back remains straight. Now straighten the legs by placing the heels on the floor first, then tightening your thighs. Try these deep knee bends 8 or more times in succession.

Body Awareness: To maintain balance during this exercise, don't let your buttocks stick out, but keep tucking them in as you hold your back straight. Are you feeling the thigh muscles toning?

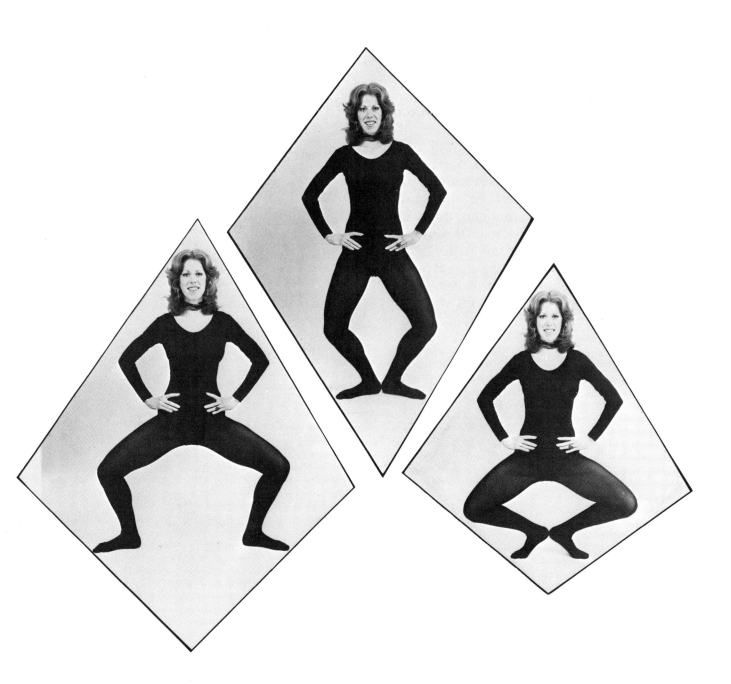

Parallel Knee Bends

Wearing platform or high-heeled shoes can cause a shortening of the heel cord and calf muscles. This easy exercise stretches the muscles and tendons in the back of the legs to prevent them from shortening or cramping. It also strengthens the thighs and helps to flatten your stomach.

Position: Stand with feet parallel and a little more than shoulder-width apart. Shrink your stomach and elongate your spine.

Start: In 4 counts, bend your knees directly over the toes as *low* as you can without lifting the heels. As the knees are bending down, raise your arms up and overhead, passing close to the ears. Stay bent and do 16 short bounces without leaning the upper body forward and without lifting the heels. Feel your weight more toward the front of the feet when bouncing. Straighten up on 4 counts while you lower the arms. Repeat the exercise (bend, bounce, straighten) for 4–6 times without pausing.

Now place one foot directly in front of the other, a pace ahead of it, and perform the beginner exercise 3 or more times without pausing. Change foot positions and repeat 3 times.

Body Awareness: When you bend, try to keep your back straight without letting the buttocks stick out. By concentrating on flattening the stomach and lifting the chest, you can avoid collapsing your weight onto the bent knees. Are you feeling the tendons and calf muscles stretching? You may also be feeling the front thighs building strength.

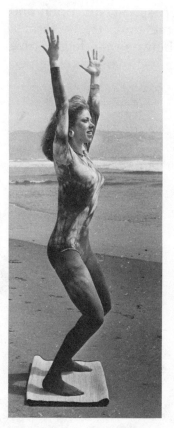 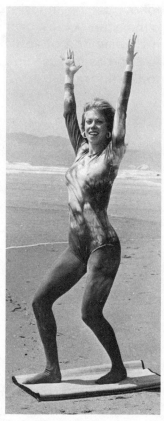

Balletic Knee Bends

One of the most strenuous of all physical activities is the graceful art of ballet dancing. This basic ballet exercise (usually done at the barre) strengthens and tones the thighs and buttocks. These knee bends are often used as a warm-up exercise for the legs.

Position: Stand sideways to a wall (or support) and place one hand on it. Place one foot directly in front of you, and turn it so the heel faces center and the toes turn outward. Now place the other foot right in front of it and turn it in the opposite direction. Bend your knees and try to make the heel of one foot touch the toes of the other.

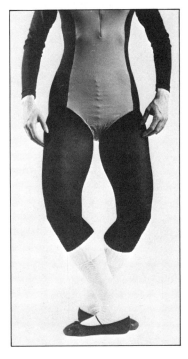

This is the fifth position in ballet. The hardest part about this position is in aligning your feet so they touch, heels to toes. If your feet won't turn out enough, they'll leave a space between toes and heels. Don't worry about it. Keep trying to close the space.

Beginners: Straighten your knees without altering the foot position. Now slowly bend your knees wide over the toes in 2 counts. Bend them as low as you can without lifting your heels or leaning your upper body forward. Stay low and bounce them very gently for 2 counts, then straighten the legs on 2 counts. Repeat the set: bend for 2, bounce 2, straighten 2. Perform 10 sets, then switch feet and repeat. Remember to bend the knees as low as you can without lifting the heels.

Intermediates: Follow the beginner exercise without touching a support. After you straighten your knees, press up on to the balls of your feet and balance for 2 counts.

Advanced: Follow the intermediate exercise. After you've balanced for 2 counts on the balls of your feet, return your heels to the floor then do a deep knee-bend without moving the foot position. As you bend, open your knees wide over your toes and keep your heels touching. Straighten up by letting your heels touch the floor first, as in the photo. Try 10 sets, adding the deep knee bend, then switch feet for 10.

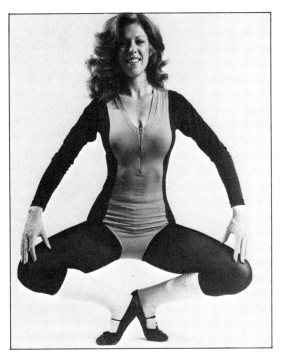

Body Awareness: Aside from the fifth position of the feet, the most difficult part of this exercise is in keeping your back straight and your bottom tucked under (don't let it stick out in back when you bend your knees). Are you really feeling your thighs and buttocks building strength?

The Lean

To contour front thigh muscles.

Position: On your knees with legs together or a few inches apart. Arms reach forward. Straighten your back and flatten the stomach. Draw the buttock muscles together.

Beginners: Lean backward in 4 slow counts, keeping the back straight. Come up in 4 counts and relax. Repeat 3 more times, trying to lean farther back each time.

Intermediates and Advanced: Follow the beginner version, leaning as far back as possible with the upper body so that it is cutting a long diagonal line. Hold the long lean position 4–8 counts, then straighten up on 4 counts. Repeat at least twice or more.

Body Awareness: Try not to release the buttocks and hips into a "sitting" position—tuck them under as you lean back. Keep lengthening the back, reaching out through the top of your head. Do you feel those thigh muscles building strength?

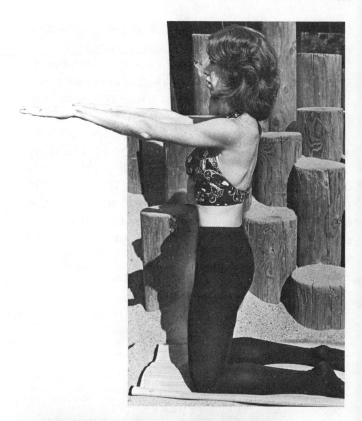

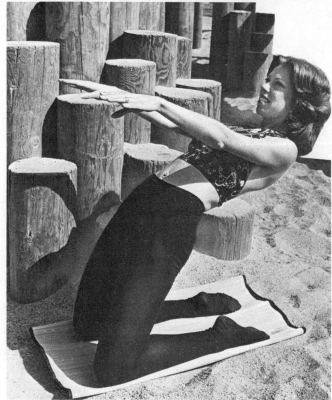

The Holdout

To contour and strengthen the thighs, try this control-and-balance challenge.

Position: Stand with your stomach contracted, chest elevated, and back lengthened. Press the shoulder tips down. Extend your left arm sideways and brace the hand against a support. Now raise your right knee sideways, close to your right waist, and grasp it with the right hand. Straighten the left knee by pulling up hard from the kneecap.

Beginners: Bounce the right knee up to your right waist 4 times with toes pointed. Release your grip on the knee and straighten the leg out to the side. It's okay to let the leg drop in height so that it is at a diagonal (45-degree angle) from your hip. Hold the leg sideways in the air for 4 slow counts as you point your toes and straighten the knee hard. Now bend the knee up to your side again and grasp it with the right hand. Repeat the set 3 or 4 times before you relax the leg to

the floor. Change sides and repeat the sets with the left leg. If stamina permits, try the sequence again on each side.

Intermediates and advanced: Follow the beginner sets except: Do not use a support when bouncing your knee up to the side. Also, when you straighten the leg sideways, try to hold it up in the air a little higher. Hold it up for 8 counts instead of 4.

Now copy the beginner sets without using a support. When you straighten the leg to the side, hold it for 8 counts at waist level (or higher!).

Body Awareness: Think of keeping your back and the standing leg very straight. You're cheating if you tip forward or sideways. By not letting your upper body collapse or your hips twist, you can maintain balance. No doubt you are feeling those top thigh muscles toning!

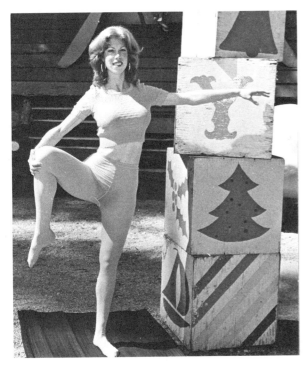
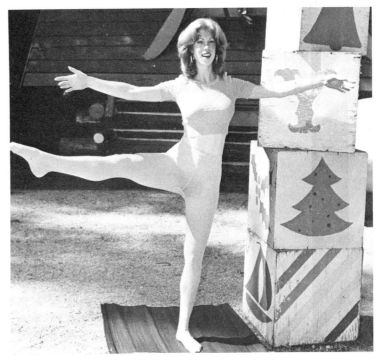

Seated Sidekicks

For buttocks, upper thighs, and hips in need of toning, try this seated sidekick.

Position: Side-sit with right leg folded in front, heel to crotch, and left leg folded to the side, heel to buttock. Try to sit squarely on both buttocks. Lengthen your back. You may feel a stretch along the top of the left thigh in this position.

Beginners: Grasp your right leg with both hands. Raise just your left buttock off the floor and hold it up for 4 counts. Now raise the left leg off the floor a few inches (keep the knee bent) and hold it up for 4 slow beats. Lower the leg and repeat 2 or 3 more times.

Change sides so that the left leg is bent front and the right leg is folded to the side. Repeat on the second side 2 or 3 times.

Intermediates: Follow the beginner exercise with your arms extended out to the sides. When you are in the side-sit position, both buttocks and both knees should be touching the floor.

Advanced: Side-sit with your arms extended. Lift the left leg off the floor a few inches and hold it up for 4 beats. Now straighten the left leg sideways in the air and hold it for 4 more counts. Keeping it straight, kick it up gently 4 times. Then fold it in on 4 counts and set it down. Repeat the set twice more. Change sides and do 3 more sets.

Body Awareness: When you raise your left leg, try not to lean too far over to the right. Work at straightening your back.

You may feel a cramp in the lifted buttock, a sign of muscle weakness from disuse. If a cramp occurs, set the leg down and pound out the cramp gently with your fists. As you practice this exercise, cramps will decrease. Feel the buttock and upper-thigh muscles toning?

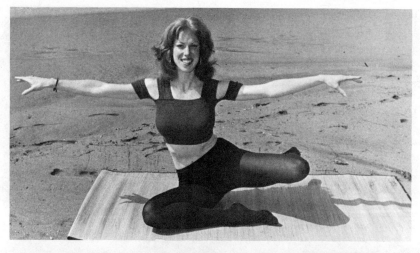

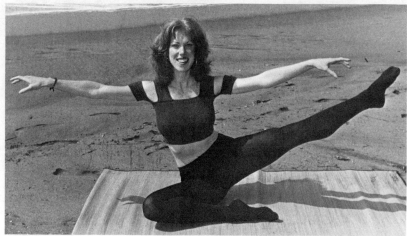

Folded Kick-ups

If your goal is stronger, firmer thighs, then try these challenging swift kicks.

Position: Sit in a half-split position: One leg is stretched out to the side, toes pointed; the other leg is folded, heel to buttock. Place both hands on the floor, one in front of you and the other to the side. Straighten your spine. You should be feeling an inner-thigh stretch in this position.

Beginners: Without leaning back, kick the straight leg up and down for 8 counts. Raise it only a few inches off the floor when you kick. On the 8th count, hold the leg up for 4 slow counts before lowering it to the floor. Repeat twice more, then change leg positions for 3 sets. If stamina permits, try the sequence again.

Intermediates: Follow the beginner exercise with your arms extended out to the sides. Try not to lean back when you kick.

Advanced: Follow the intermediate version with your arms stretched overhead. Throw your leg up high 8 times, then hold it high without letting it drop in height for 8. Repeat the sets 3 times on each side, alternating legs.

Body Awareness: You'll need to lean back slightly, but you're actually cheating if you lean way back every time you kick. Try to keep your spine straight throughout the exercise. Are you feeling the front thigh muscles building strength?

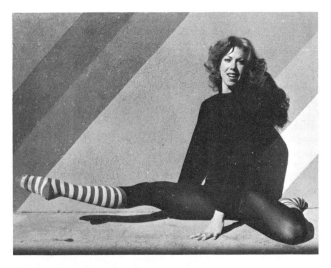

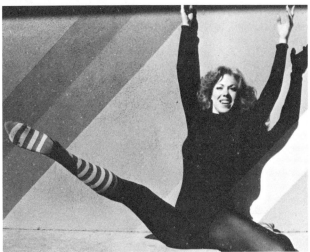

Balanced Foldout

Here's a challenging balancing act that also strengthens your hip and thigh muscles.

Position: Squat down and place your hands on the floor.

Beginners: Lift one thigh as high as you can to the side, with your knee bent, and hold it up for 12 slow counts. Now raise one arm to the side and try to balance for 4–8 counts without letting your thigh drop in height! Lower the arm and leg and change sides. Repeat the set 2 more times.

Intermediates: Perform one set of the beginner exercise with each leg. Perform the next two sets with your lifted leg held straight out to the side.

Bending that knee is cheating.

Advanced: Follow the intermediate version by holding your leg straight out to the side for 12 counts. Now keep your leg up, point your toes, spread your arms sideways, smile, and balance for 4–8 counts. Try 2–3 sets on each side.

Body Awareness: The key is to lift the weight of your upper torso out of your hips, rather than letting your weight collapse down and forward onto your knees. If you start to feel too much pressure on your knees and you're not collapsing your weight onto them, then don't continue the exercise.

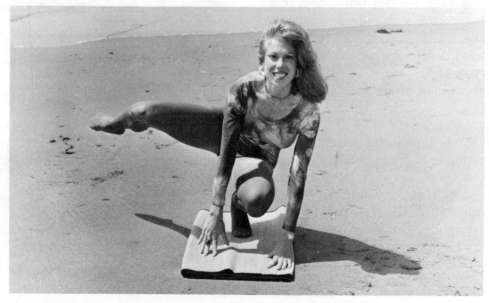

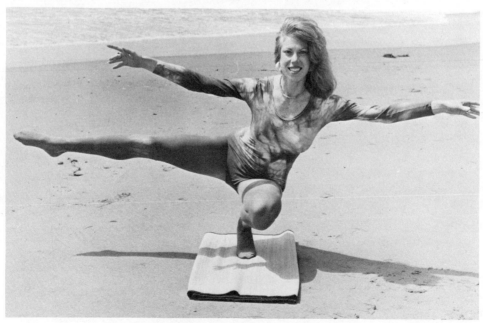

Single Leg Raises

Tone and shape the front thighs while stretching muscles in the back of the thighs.

Position: Sit with your upper back against a wall, hips and lower back a few inches away from it. Bend your knees up so the feet are flat on the floor close to your buttocks. Hands are on the floor at your sides.

Beginners: In 4 counts, straighten one leg up in the air as high as possible. Hold it up for 8 slow counts with the knee kept very straight and the toes pointed. Bend the leg in on 4. Repeat before changing legs. Continue by alternating legs every second set for 8–12 sets (or as long as stamina permits). As your leg strength improves, try holding the leg up for 12 counts.

Intermediates and Advanced: Assume the beginner position, except stretch your arms out to the sides. Perform 4 sets in this position. Now scoot forward slightly so your back doesn't touch the wall, and repeat the exercise for 4–8 more sets.

Body Awareness: You may feel a terrific pull up the back of your thigh when you try to straighten a leg. If these thigh muscles are inflexible, they will prevent you from raising the leg high. The main idea in this exercise is to keep the knee very straight at whatever height your flexibility permits. In the advanced version you'll also feel the stomach muscles working.

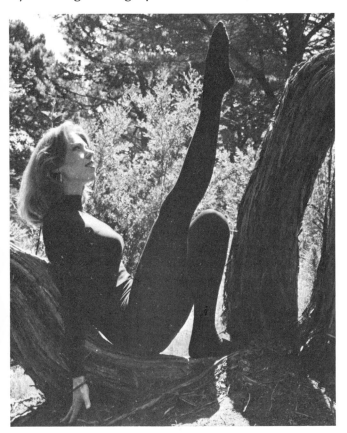

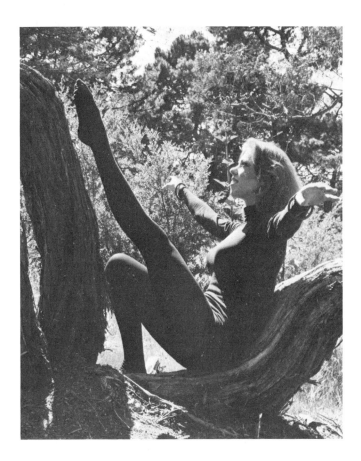

Double Leg Raises

A strengthener for weak thigh and stomach muscles.

Position: Sit so that you are leaning back onto your forearms with your knees bent up to your chest.

Beginners: In 4 slow counts, slowly straighten both legs up to the ceiling. Hold them up for 12 counts with the toes pointed and the knees kept very straight. Now bend the knees on 4 and return to starting position. Continue straightening, holding, bending without pausing for at least 6 sets. Increase the sets as stamina permits. When the legs straighten in the air, try to lift some of your body weight off of the forearms. By drawing the shoulder blades together in back, you can keep from collapsing onto your forearms while the legs straighten.

Intermediates: Follow the beginner version, sitting up higher so that you are bracing yourself on just your hands. The arms are very straight (no bent elbows) during the exercise.

Advanced: Alter the starting position so that you are sitting with your arms wrapped around the knees. Straighten the legs *and* arms in the air on 4 counts so that you are balancing on just your buttocks. Now grasp both ankles and hold your head to the knees for 8 counts. Return to starting position (4 counts) and repeat for 6 or more sets. The key here is not to lose your balance. If you let your back round too much, you'll roll backward.

Body Awareness: For maximum benefit, deflate your stomach every time the legs straighten in the air. Be sure the knees don't bend during the hold. Are you feeling the front thighs and the stomach muscles toning?

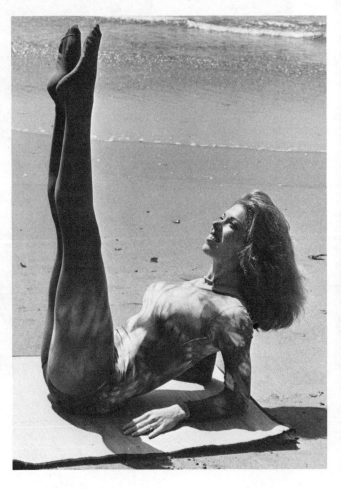
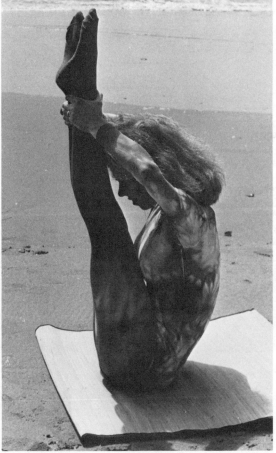

Fulcrum

Challenge your balance as you strengthen the thighs and stretch your waist.

Position: Stand with your weight on the left leg. The left hand is grasping the side of your left thigh. Stretch your right arm overhead close to your ear. Now draw the stomach in and elongate your entire body.

Beginners: Take 4 counts to lift the right leg sideways a few inches (or higher if possible) so you are cutting a diagonal line in space with your body. Hold for 8 counts without losing balance. Lower the arm and leg on 4, then repeat before changing sides. Continue the exercise 4–6 times, alternating sides every second set.

Intermediates: Follow the beginner exercise, except raise the leg up higher as you tilt your upper body farther. Balance-hold for 8 counts before straightening up on 4. Repeat 4–6 times, changing sides every second set.

Advanced: From starting position, raise your left leg as high as possible while you lean over slowly to the right. Take as many counts as you need to adjust your balance. Continue leaning and lifting the leg until you are stretched out from toes to fingertips along a straight, horizontal plane. Balance-hold for 8 counts, then straighten up on 4 counts. Repeat then change sides. Try the set once or twice more.

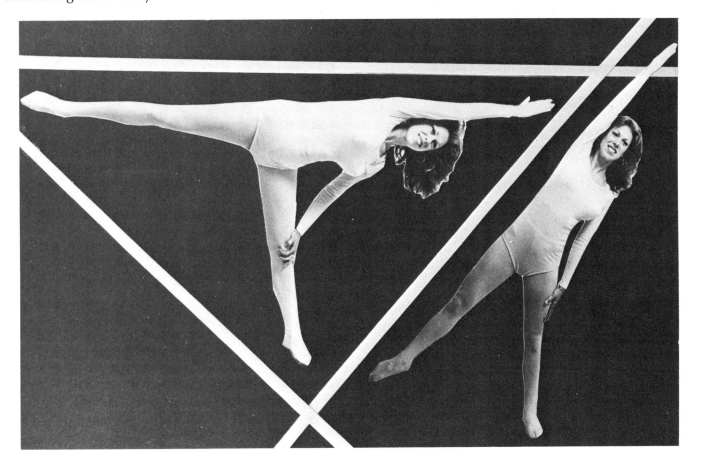

Body Awareness: Imagine that strings are attached to your fingertips and to the toes of the lifted leg. As you lean and balance, feel an equal but opposite pull on the strings to help stretch you long. Holding your stomach in will aid your balance. My beginners wobble and lose balance at first. With practice, especially before a mirror, balance gradually improves. Do you feel the thigh muscles building strength?

Mini-Lifter

Surprisingly enough, some of the easiest muscles to custom-contour are the front thigh muscles. This exercise serves a dual purpose, as you'll be toning the thighs and stomach muscles simultaneously.

Position: Sit up very straight on the floor with your legs extended and together, toes pointed. If just sitting straight in this position causes a strain on your back or feels difficult, then lean up against a wall with your hips flush up against it for support.

Beginners and Intermediates: Place your hands palms down on the floor alongside your thighs. To do this, you'll need to lean forward slightly, but keep your back straight. Lift one leg a few inches off the floor and hold it up for 4 counts with the toes pointed. Now flex the foot by pushing through the heel, and hold it there for another 4 counts. Lower the leg, then repeat without pausing. Do the point-flex set twice with your other leg. Repeat the sets twice on each side for 6–8 times.

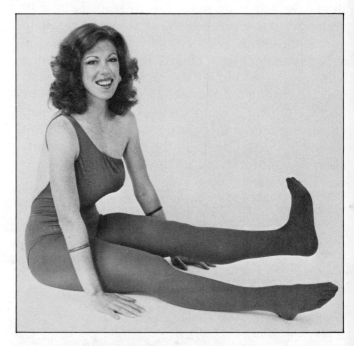

Now, without using a wall for support, try the exercise with your hands placed next to your knees. Remember to keep your back straight, and don't let your shoulders round. This time, do 3 sets of the point (4 counts)–and–flex (4 counts) combination with one leg, before changing to the other. Repeat the sets 8 or more times.

Advanced: Follow the intermediate instructions by performing 3 sets of the point-flex combination with the right, then the left leg. Now press down hard with both hands and lift *both* legs a few inches off the floor simultaneously! Try to hold them up for 4–8 counts before lowering. Repeat the exercise 2–3 more times without pausing.

Body Awareness: You're cheating if you lean back even a little when you lift a leg. Pull your stomach in and keep your knees very straight. Expect to feel the front thigh muscles working! Depending upon your flexibility, you may also be feeling the back thigh and lower back muscles stretching.

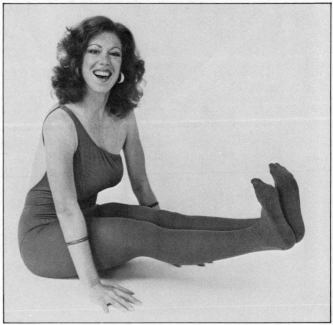

Mini-Lifter Variation

Spot exercises, the right and wrong way: There is a right and a wrong way to perform every exercise, and if you are not shown the correct way, you could be wasting your time (or, even worse, harming your body).

Here is one exercise that tones the stomach and thighs simultaneously, but if performed incorrectly won't do a thing for you.

Position: Sit alongside a wall with your legs together, knees straight and toes pointed. Lengthen and straighten your back to its utmost, then raise one hand overhead and touch the wall. If sitting up straight without support causes discomfort in your back, alter the position so that your hips and back are flush up against the wall.

The Right Way: Keeping your back very straight, draw your stomach in and raise one leg a few inches off the floor. Hold the leg up for 3 slow counts; set it down on the 4th count. Repeat for 8–10 times (or more, depending on your stamina), then change legs and repeat. Try the set once more. Turn around, raise your other hand overhead against the wall, and perform the set once or twice again.

The Wrong Way: You'll lose all the good benefits of this exercise if you lean backward, if you let your stomach pop out, or if you round your shoulders. By cheating the exercise as in this photo, you may be able to lift your legs higher, but you won't be helping the stomach or thighs. Are you also feeling your lower and upper back muscles stretching?

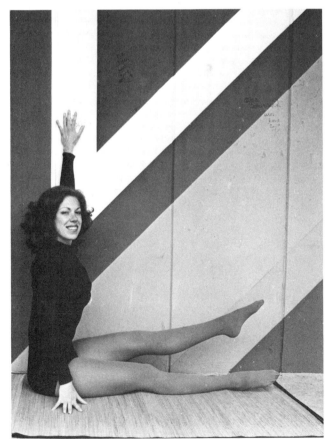
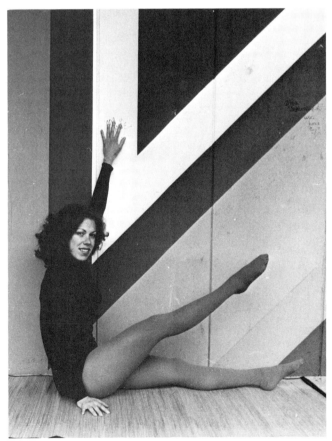

The Scissors

To strengthen the stomach and tone the thighs.

Position: Lie on your back with legs extended straight up, heels together and toes pointed. Extend arms out to the sides. Press the small of your back into the floor.

Beginners: Slowly spread the legs wide apart in 4 counts, keeping the knees very straight. Bring them together on 4. Relax by bending the legs to your chest. Straighten them up again on 4 and repeat the Scissors. Try the set 3–6 times, bending the knees to the chest between each set.

Intermediates and Advanced: Take 4 counts to open the legs, hold them open for 4, then bring them together on 4. Continue the set 4–8 times (or until strength is depleted) without pausing and without bending the knees.

Body Awareness: Constantly draw the stomach in and keep the shoulders on the floor while the legs are working. Feel the stomach and leg muscles building strength!

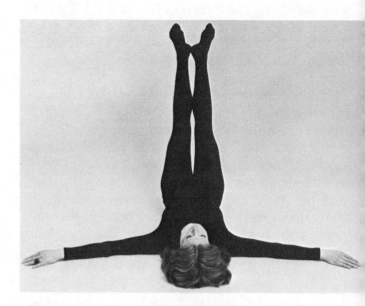

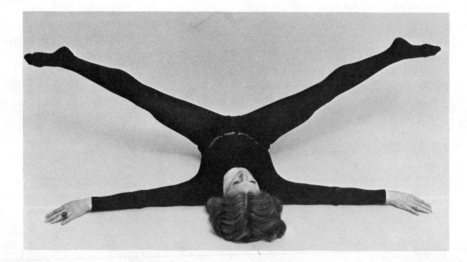

Barbell Squat

Traditionally, weight-lifting for women has been taboo. Women watched men on a weight-lifting program slowly develop bulging biceps and concluded that the muscular look was not the desired body image for any female.

Actually, weight training (or resistance exercises, as it is also called) is the most efficient way to strengthen and contour the figure. Those mounds of muscles that men develop from intensive weight lifting are the result of the body's secretion of testosterone, the male hormone.

Women also secrete this hormone, but in much smaller amounts, thereby preventing them from ever developing bulky, blown-up muscles. Women can streamline, strengthen, and contour their figures more efficiently and effectively with weight-lifting exercises than with traditional calisthenics.

But if the contouring results from weight lifting are so effective, why do so many women resist (pardon the pun) using weights? The main complaint is that weight lifting doesn't provide the aesthetic, free, joyous experience that an excellent no-weights exercise program can and should provide.

Ultimately, if you're not enjoying the workout sessions, (weight-lifting or otherwise) your good intentions and initial efforts will wane before you attain the desired results.

This exercise, called half-squats or deep knee bends, is done with a barbell to add extra resistance for the thigh muscles. The easiest way of determining the correct amount of weight for you is the old-fashioned trial-and-error method. Pick a weight you can handle without too much strain to complete the specified number of sets and repetitions. If you can't complete the program, the weight is too heavy. A suggested starting weight is 15–20 pounds.

Position: Stand with your feet about shoulder-width apart and bend your arms up near your shoulders, palms toward the ceiling.

Beginners: Have someone place the barbell on your shoulders behind your neck. With your back straight, lower the weight by bending your knees halfway as if you were taking a seat. Return to standing position by slowly straightening your knees. Repeat the half-squats a total of 15–20 times without pausing.

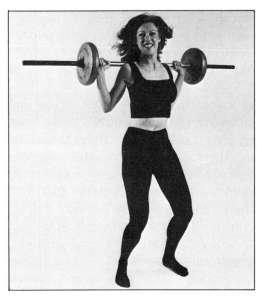

Intermediates: Follow the beginner version, except do one set of 15 half-squats, pause for a minute, then do a second set of 15. Gradually increase the amount of weight when the exercise becomes easier for you to accomplish.

Advanced: Squat all the way down without letting your back sway. When you straighten up from the full squat position, immediately place your heels flat on the floor, then straighten your knees completely. You should be using heavier weights, and you should be striving to do 3 sets of 5–10 repetitions per set (with a minute or less pause between sets).

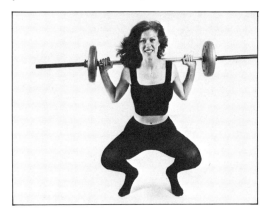

Body Awareness: In order to achieve strength and contour in the thighs, you'll need to increase the amount of weight (resistance) once you can easily complete the designated number of sets. Try to keep your stomach in and your shoulders straight, not rounded.

Leg Fan

Double strength, double stretch: Here's a four-way exercise—it strengthens your thighs and stomach while it stretches your waist and back.

Position: Lie on your back on the floor, arms at your sides.

Beginners: Raise the left leg skyward in four counts (let both knees bend a little). Cross your left leg over your body to the right side, and lower it to the floor. You're striving to touch the left toes to the right hand, or as close as possible (4 counts). Hold for 8 beats with your head turned away from the crossed leg. Slowly lower the leg down and return to starting position (4 beats). Continue the set without a pause for 8–16 times, then change legs and repeat. The leg should move in a smooth, continuous flow as it raises, crosses, and lowers.

Intermediates: Follow the beginner exercise for 4 sets without bending either knee. For the next 4 sets, raise one leg skyward, cross it to the opposite side, then continue circling it down, around to the other side, straight up, across, etc., so you are describing huge circles with your leg. Slowly circle the leg 8 times before changing sides.

Advanced: Follow the intermediate exercise with both legs glued tightly together as if they were one. Circle them around slowly 4 times in one direction, then 4 in the other. Pause. Repeat the set of 8 circles.

Body Awareness: My beginning students tend to let their shoulders and lower back creep up off the floor during the exercise. For maximum results, try to keep your hips and entire spine pressed to the floor. Are you feeling the thighs and stomach building strength? You should also be feeling the waist and back stretching.

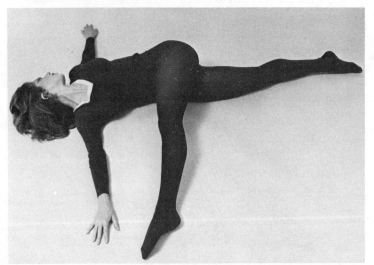
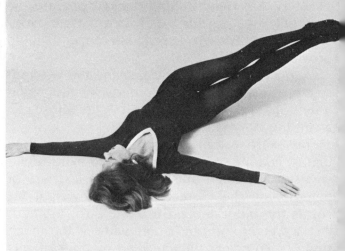

Flutter Kicks

You can contour your thighs at the same time that you firm your stomach with these flutter kicks.

Position: Lie back onto your elbows and forearms and straighten your legs skyward with toes pointed. Cross one leg over the other.

Beginners: In 12 animated counts, crisscross your legs back and forth. Lower them gradually toward the floor during the first set of 6 crosses, and raise them for the second set of 6. Now bend the knees to your chest for 2 counts to relax the legs. Straighten them skyward again and repeat the exercise in a continuous flutter of leg crosses down and up. Continue the exercise 3 more times (or more if stamina permits).

Intermediates: Perform 2 sets of the beginner exercise. Now place your palms on the floor slightly behind your hips and perform 4 sets of the same exercise supported on your hands instead of on your elbows and forearms.

Advanced: For openers, perform 2 beginner, then 2 intermediate sets. Now reach your arms up and perform the same exercise 3 times while you are balancing on your buttocks. Your legs should become a flutter of crosses on the descent and ascent.

Body Awareness: You're cheating if your knees bend. Keep the legs pulled straight and taut, and remember to draw your stomach in while your legs are fluttering about. Are you feeling the front thighs and stomach muscles building strength?

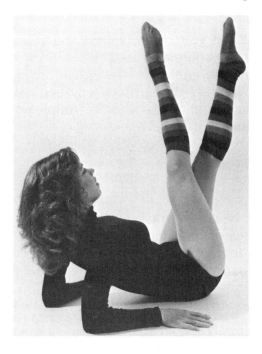 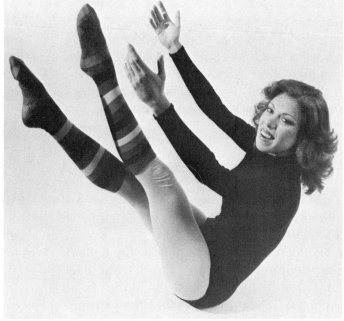

Ski with Mops I

Even if you don't ski, the following three exercises will tone your thighs.

Whether it's downhill racing or cross-country skiing, you'll have a safer, easier time of it with some preseason conditioning. And you don't have to own any fancy ski equipment in order to practice warming up before you hit the slopes. A couple of household mops can substitute very nicely for ski poles.

Position: Stand your mops a little more than shoulder-width apart with the handles straight up. Grasp the "poles" near the top and extend your arms straight out in front of you. Now place one leg forward and the other stretched as far behind it as you can, keeping your heels on the floor. Draw your stomach in gently.

Start: Bend forward from your hips as far as you can while keeping your back very straight. Hold the position for 12 counts. Now drop your back knee almost to the floor, lift the back heel,

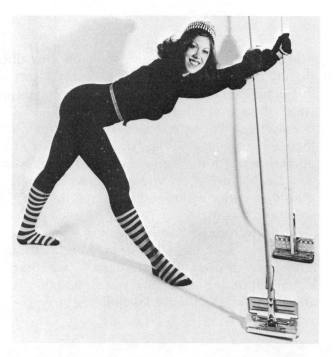

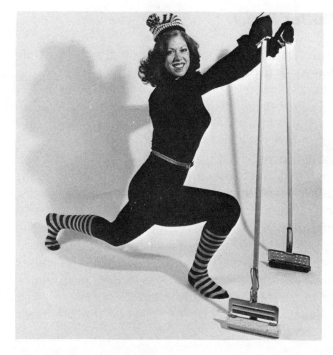

and bend the front knee over the toes. Stretch your arms farther so that your hands reach the top of your "poles." Keeping your back straight, gently bounce your back knee up and down, close to the floor, 12 times. Straighten both legs again and repeat the sequence by bending for-

ward from your hips first. If stamina permits, repeat the entire exercise.

Body Awareness: This is a great pre-ski conditioner because it helps to strengthen and stretch the thighs and calves, muscle groups most apt to tire quickly on the slopes.

Ski with Mops II

Position: Grasp your "poles" gently, squeeze your buttocks tightly together, draw your stomach in, and straighten your back.

Start: In 4 counts, rise up high onto the balls of your feet. Keeping your heels lifted, your back very straight, and your stomach sucked in, bend your knees just a few inches. Hold the "sitting" position for 8 counts. You're cheating if you let your buttocks stick out too far in back when the knees are bent (try to keep them tucked under). Now straighten your knees in 4 counts, then lower your heels on 4. Repeat the sequence at least 6 times, each time bending your knees a little more so that you're "sitting" closer to the ground.

Now lift one foot a few inches off the floor and try the same exercise 4 times, balancing on one foot only, then four times on the other foot. Do you wobble too much when you're on one foot? If so, your feet or thighs may be weak, or you might be collapsing your upper body when you try to balance.

Body Awareness: Since balance as well as thigh strength are vital to skillful skiing, this exercise

would be worth practicing daily. Try not to lean too dependently on your "poles"; grasp them gently so you can train your body to be in control and balance with little need for external support.

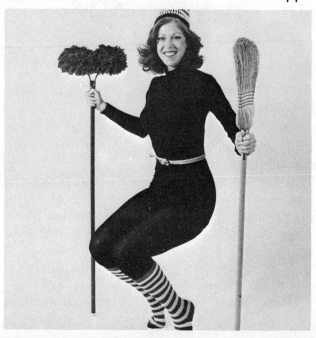

Snowplow

The "snowplow" position (feet turned in) is one way to stop yourself while skiing. This exercise uses the snowplow position to help prevent shin splints and build strength in your thighs.

Position: Stand with your feet placed about shoulder-width apart and toes turned in to face each other. Touch a wall or any support with your back or hand.

Beginners: In 4 counts, bend your knees over the toes until the knees knock together and form a triangle of space below them. Don't let your heels leave the floor. Gently bounce the knees down and toward each other for 4 counts, then straighten them on 4. Repeat the set 6–8 times or more. Be sure knees bend directly over toes, not in front of them.

Intermediates: Stand in the above position with your heels lifted high so that your weight is on the toes and balls of the feet. Now follow the beginner exercise with your heels up.

Advanced: Perform one set of the intermediate exercise. For the second set, bend the knees all the way to a squat position, keeping the knees touching throughout. Continue alternating sets 6–8 times.

Body Awareness: You're cheating if you lean forward or if you let your rear protrude when you bend. Keep your toes turned in as much as possible throughout the exercise. In the beginner version you should be feeling the lower leg and foot muscles stretching. Intermediates and advanced should also feel the feet and thighs strengthening.

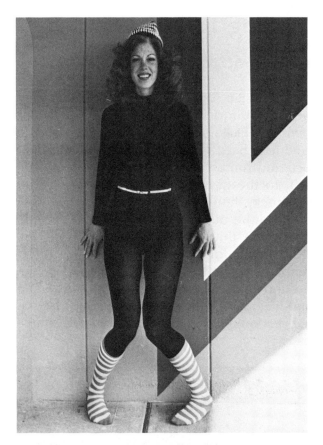

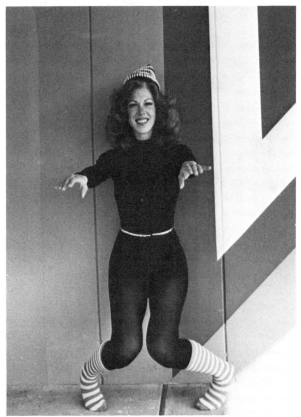

Stretching Technique

Easy Thigh-Stretcher

Position: Kneel with your legs together, then sit back with buttocks on your heels.

Beginners: Place palms flat on the floor next to feet and lean back slightly. Now lift just the right buttock and hip a few inches off the heel then touch it to the heel again. Repeat 4 times with right buttock, then with the left one.

Each time the buttock and hip lift, you should feel the front thigh muscles stretch. Continue without pausing for 4–8 sets.

Intermediates: Follow the beginner version, but place hands and forearms on the floor so that you are leaning farther back. In this and the advanced version, you might also feel an abdominal stretch.

Advanced: Slowly lean all the way back so that your upper back and head are on the floor. Hold that position for 12 or more counts before sitting up. Repeat, staying down for as long as you can.

Body Awareness: If you're feeling pressure along the front of your feet, you're probably letting your upper-body weight collapse onto them. To correct this, draw in stomach, tuck bottom under, and lean way back so that less weight is on the feet.

Try to keep your knees together. The farther back you lean, the more they'll want to separate. Are you aware of the front thigh muscles stretching?

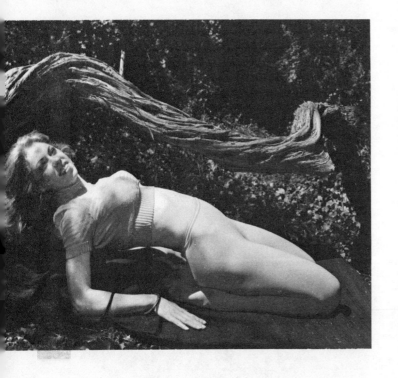
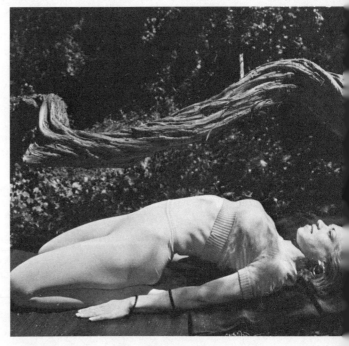

Kneeling Thigh Stretch

After a few hours of most any sport, the front thigh muscles can become stiff. Here's a good way to loosen them.

Position: Get down on your left knee and place a cushion under it. Put your right foot flat on the floor about three paces ahead of your left knee. Now slide the left knee back a little so your weight is more toward the thigh than the knee.

Beginners: Touch a wall or support with your right hand and raise your left foot off the floor, grasping it from behind with your left hand. Pull-bounce your foot toward the left buttock 8 times. While you're still holding your foot, lean forward toward the right leg (keep your back straight) and hold the position for 8 counts. Change legs and repeat. Try the set at least once more on both sides.

Intermediates: Perform one set of the beginner exercise. After you bounce forward for 8 counts, arch back and aim the top of your head toward the left foot. Hold for 8 counts then change legs and repeat.

Advanced: Follow the intermediate exercise but hold your back foot up with *both* hands when you arch backward. In this position you're also testing your balance!

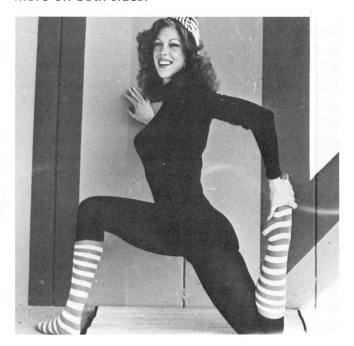 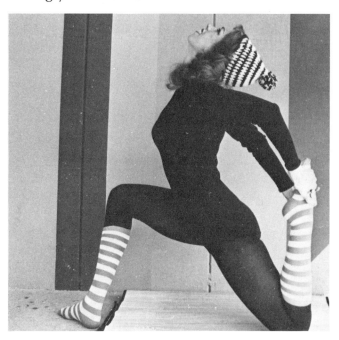

Body Awareness: When you arch backward, try to lift your chest high while you pull your foot toward your buttock. Are you feeling a super-stretch along the back thigh?

Folded Thigh Stretch

Here's a superstretch for the front thigh muscles.

Position: Sit with your right leg folded front, heel to crotch; left leg folded to the side, heel to buttock. Try to sit on both buttocks with both knees on the floor. Just sitting in this position may in itself produce a stretch along your front thigh muscles. Elongate your back.

Beginners: Place your hands on the floor behind you, a comfortable distance away with the elbows straight. In 4 slow counts, bend the elbows so you are leaning back to the point that your thigh muscles have reached their stretch limit. Hold back for 8–12 counts, then straighten the elbows on 4. Repeat slowly for 6–8 continuous sets.

Intermediates: Follow the beginner exercise, except: lean farther back so your weight is on your forearms and elbows. Hold the position for 12 counts before straightening the elbows on 4. Repeat 6–8 times.

Advanced: In 4 slow counts, lower your back all the way down to the floor with your arms on the floor at your sides. Hold the position for 12 counts, then sit up on 4. Repeat the set 4 times without pausing.

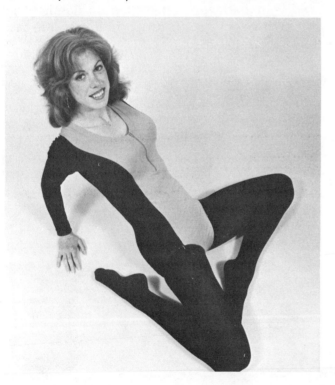

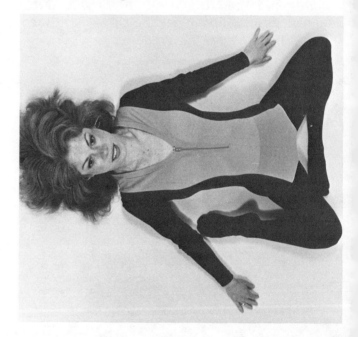

Body Awareness: If one buttock or knee creeps up off the floor, then you are cheating! Are you feeling those front thigh muscles stretching?

Sprinter

Whether you run, jog, dance, ski, or whatever, this is one good warm-up exercise that works your heart muscle while it stretches your inner thighs for maximum extension.

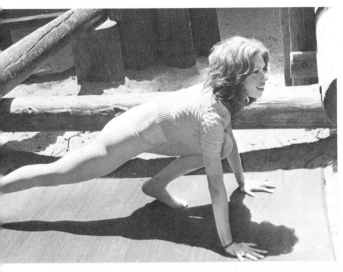

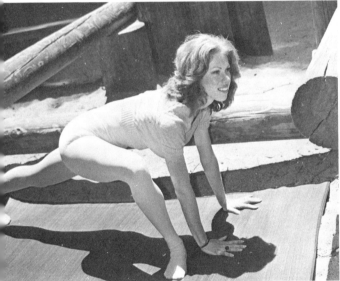

Position: Get down on all fours with your left leg extended straight back and your right knee bent over your toes. Lift both heels. Your back should be straight and your head lifted.

Start: Complete 4 lively bounces up and down with your back knee pulled straight. Now immediately jump-switch your legs and repeat. Continue bouncing for 4 counts, then jump-switch legs without a pause for 4 sets, or as long as stamina permits.

Each day try to increase the number of sets so that you can do at least 8 bounces before switching legs. Then do 4 sets in succession without pausing.

Variation: Bounce 4 times with your right knee bent forward and toes straight ahead. Now turn the right foot so that your toes face out, heel to center, and your right foot is flat on the floor. Bounce 4 more times, then quickly jump-switch legs and repeat on the other side (4 bounces with toes straight; 4 with them turned out). Repeat the set at least 3 more times, alternating legs without pausing.

Body Awareness: As you bounce, keep your head up and your back flat and elongated. You should feel the stretch mostly along your inner and outer thighs and at the buttocks.

Sidesprint

A long stretch to restore resiliency to stiff inner thighs.

Position: Stand with feet wide apart and toes parallel. Bend both knees and place both hands on the floor. Flatten your back so it is parallel with the floor, and keep the head up.

Beginners: Bounce your bottom up and down 4 times in the above position, letting your knees bend and straighten slightly as you bounce. Keep your hands flat on the floor. Now try to straighten just your right knee (be careful), and bend your left knee low over the left toes. Stop at the point where you feel a pull along the inner thighs. Bounce 4 times in this lunge position. Change legs so that the left knee is straight and the right knee is bent directly over the toes. Bounce 4 times, then return to center with both knees bent. Repeat the lunge-bounce combination in each direction for 6–8 rounds. Count very slowly, don't rush yourself while you bounce.

Intermediates: Assume a longer, wider lunge, with one leg completely straight while the other knee is bent low over the toes. Follow the beginner exercise, bouncing 8 times in each of 3 directions for 6–8 rounds, or as stamina permits.

Advanced: After bouncing 8 times, stay low and hold the position for 4 slow beats. Repeat the set before you change the direction of your lunge. Continue bouncing and holding low for 4–6 rounds, changing direction after every second set.

Body Awareness: Don't let either foot lift off the floor when you lunge-bounce sideways. You can prevent rounded, tense shoulders by keeping your head up and your back flat. Feel the inner-thigh and buttock muscles stretch as the front thigh muscles are building strength? I strongly advise beginning students not to attempt too wide a lunge at first. Eventually, by practicing the sidesprint daily, the thigh muscles will thaw and grow more resilient.

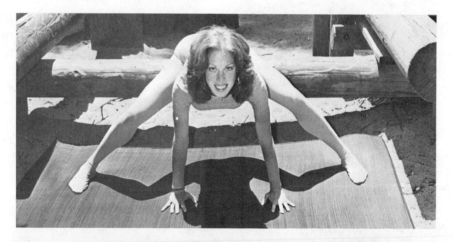

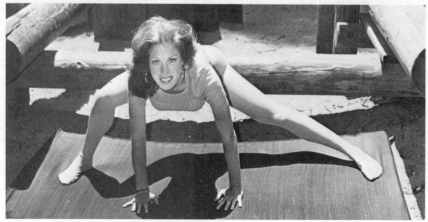

Eastern Split

Traditionally, the martial arts were considered a group of disciplines that one studied for the sole purpose of self-defense. These days many peace-loving men, women, and children are learning the various Oriental ways of weaponless self-defense for excellent overall exercise.

Here is one exercise borrowed from karate that helps keep the inner thighs supple, thereby allowing you those high kicks and long strides that are also important to many other sports.

Position: Stand with your feet wide apart, toes facing forward and knees bent. Lean over and place your fingertips on the floor in front of you.

Beginners: Bend just your right knee over the toes as you straighten the left knee completely. Keep both feet flat, still facing forward, and bounce the bent knee slightly up and down 4 times. Now try to stay close to the floor and hold the bent-knee position for 4 counts. Repeat the bounce-hold. Straighten the right leg. Lean over to the left side, letting the left knee bend over the toes, and straighten the right leg sideways. Bounce 4; hold 4; repeat; then straighten the left knee. Repeat the entire set 3 more times.

Intermediates: Follow the beginner exercise. You should be able to bounce-hold while staying low to the floor. Repeat the sequence 3 times with the right knee bent, then 3 times with the left knee bent. Repeat the set 6 times without pausing.

Advanced: Perform one or two of the intermediate sets. Now straighten both legs, lean forward, and very slowly and carefully let the legs split apart until the calves and inner thighs are touching the floor. Hold the position for 16 counts. Relax, then repeat.

Body Awareness: For maximum stretch benefit, always keep one knee completely straight. If you find it too difficult to perform this exercise with your weight on the fingertips, then flatten your palms on the floor. Be sure you're being gentle at the same time that you're feeling an inner-thigh stretch.

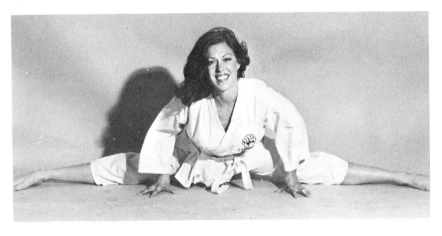

Secret Thigh Exercises

● Since the thigh muscles are stronger than the back muscles, the former should do the heavy lifting. Squat all the way down and close to a heavy object, and lift it with your back held completely straight. Now the thighs can do the main work.

● Bend your knees deeply to reach an item on a lower shelf, then straighten up *without* leaning forward or holding on to anything for support.

● When you get into or out of a chair, don't depend on the arm rests for help. Instead, let your thigh muscles contract to lower and raise your body while your back is kept straight.

● Climb stairs two at a time, with a straight back and without leaning dependently on the handrail.

● In the theater, on a bus, or during a meeting, sit with your lower back against the chair, then press your two legs tightly together as if they were one for as long as possible.

● When you answer the phone at work, sit up in your chair, raise both legs to hip level (parallel to the floor), and hold them up while the caller speaks. Lower them when you speak.

● To increase your walking speed, take longer strides rather than shorter, quicker steps. By lengthening your pace you're using more of your thigh and hip muscles.

● Just before you retire at night, stand with your knees slightly bent and grip your pillow between them. Squeeze the pillow for 8 counts as if trying to crush it.

● Walking briskly, jogging, jumping, running, biking, climbing hills and stairs, and deep-knee-bending all strengthen the thigh muscles.

CHAPTER FIVE:

HOW TO BUILD YOUR BOSOM AND UPPER BODY

I Must Develop My Bust

In most societies the arms and chest are considered the "glamor" muscles of the body. Those smooth swells that peak between the shoulders and elbows have always represented strength and masculinity in the male body. The smooth mounds that swell from a robust, high-arched front have always been worshiped as symbols of sensuality in the female body. When well developed, the arms and chest are the flamboyant, showy muscles that often attract the greatest attention and arouse immediate interest!

Women tend to confuse development of the chest with increasing the size of the breasts. The chest muscles (pectorals) will definitely grow and expand through certain exercises, giving the upper torso greater depth and a sense of presence. Since the breasts receive their support from the underlying chest muscles, developing the pectorals lends more support to the breasts. The uplift provides a more attractive bustline and a more pronounced profile. The actual *size* of the breasts is determined by heredity. The female breasts themselves are not composed of muscle, but of fatty tissue and mammary glands, neither of which respond to direct exercise. The only way they can be firmed or increased directly is through surgery. Oversized breasts are composed of more fatty tissue, so tend to weaken the underlying chest muscles. Sometimes their size can be decreased through diet and the type of exercise that jiggles some of the tissue off. I know of women who have lost a size or two in their breasts (loss of fatty tissue) from dieting, jogging or jumping rope.

After age 25 the breasts begin to fall and weaken the pectoral muscles that support them. Often a slouched pair of shoulders cause the breasts to sag even more. By improving posture and by developing strength in the chest muscles, the dimensions of the chest can be increased and the breasts can receive the support they need!

A healthy, strong chest appears to spring forth in front of the rest of the body, giving depth and breadth to the upper torso and allowing maximum space for the heart and lungs to expand. Unfortunately, our civilized, routine living discourages the development of a full, robust chest. Our habit of rounding the shoulders and upper back depresses the ribs, caves in the chest, and gives a contracted, crippled look to the upper body. Even-

tually the sinking rib cage shrinks and stiffens the chest muscles.

It is possible to develop a full, high chest from a flat, sunken one. Exercises that make you elevate and expand your rib cage to its fullest are effective in stretching the pectoral muscles and giving a shallow chest some depth. Stretching the chest involves the kind of exercise that moves the head and shoulders backward and reaches the arms upward, sideways, or backward while the chest is lifted. Increasing the size of the chest involves exercises designed to strengthen the arms, shoulders, and chest.

Your arms are particularly important in chest development because whenever they are raised while the back is straight or arched, they stretch the chest muscles and strengthen the shoulders, thereby keeping the chest supple and expansive instead of stiff and contracted. In turn, if the chest is tight, free arm and shoulder movement is impossible.

Think of your arms as graceful branches emanating from your trunk and bending naturally at the elbows as they sway gently at your sides. Although their muscles may be steel-strong, the arms should never lose a sense of graceful flow when they are coordinated in motion.

Since the underarm muscles (triceps) are not used frequently enough in modern life, we often develop loose, flabby sacks of flesh that droop down from underneath the upper arm. Any movements that call for straightening the arms up, down, or sideways against a resistance (i.e., the floor, a wall, weights, a partner) will help firm these muscles. Any exercise that has you bend your forearms toward your upper arm against resistance will help to develop the bicep muscles of the upper arm. Strength in your forearms, wrists, hands, and fingers can be developed by practicing tightening your grip to its maximum and by lifting heavy objects with your hands.

If you really want to increase the musculature of your chest and arms, try doing progressive-resistive-type exercises using weights. Sandbags, heavy cookware, books, dumbbells, barbells—you'll find lots of household items to serve as weights. Raising and lowering the arms slowly while they are kept straight and while you hold *equal*-sized weights in both hands will build strength in the chest, back of the upper arms (triceps), and the shoulders. Holding weights while you slowly bend the forearms to the upper arm (curling) strengthens the biceps. The number of times you repeat the exercise or the amount of weight you hold is increased according to your ability and progress. Feel free to develop a progressive-resistive weight-lifting program to improve your own strength.

The exercises in this chapter are designed mostly for weaklings who are intimidated by heavy weights. After you've built some stretch and strength in your upper body (also see backward stretches, Chapter Three), try a few of the basic weight-lifting exercises. Women need not ever worry about developing bulky muscles, a characteristic of male weight lifters, because women don't have enough testosterone (male hormone) to cause the bulky musculature. As your upper body develops in size and suppleness, it will take on a more sculptured, contoured look, and you'll begin to feel more expansive!

Your Sensual Shoulders

How do you straighten a stooped society that is forced into a slump over work and during play? Modern man's and woman's most prevalent occupations (office worker, student, seamstress, etc.) contribute toward a major posture malady: rounded shoulders due to weak upper-back muscles. Even our popular sports, such as baseball, basketball, tennis, bowling, and volleyball, have us hunched over in "waiting position" or while in action. By the time we reach adulthood, our shoulders have slipped forward permanently and we find ourselves victims of the habitual hunch.

The aches and fatigue that build on the shoulders and upper back come not just from the physical strain of slumping, but from psychological tension as well. When we encounter an emotionally or physically stressful situation, our body prepares for it. The muscles tense for action—fight or flight. If we don't take action, the unresolved conflict without a physical or psychological release can keep our muscles in a tense state. Often the greatest amount of tension accumulates in the neck, and radiates to the shoulders and upper-back muscles. Learning to relax these muscles is often more difficult than building strength in them.

Your shoulder muscles can also reflect your moods. If your success sinks, the shoulders might slump; if your spirit sails, the shoulders straighten. When you're irritated, your upper torso tenses; when you're tired, it collapses. Ultimately underexercise, gravity's constant pull, and daily annoyances can weaken the shoulders, which in turn weaken and shorten the chest muscles in front. The chest becomes concave and your posture takes on the appearance of a boiled shrimp!

Uneven shoulders are usually caused by carrying with one hand more than the other, standing with the weight more on one foot than the other, or from engaging in certain occupations and sports. The asymmetry can be corrected by strengthening the muscles on the dropped side and by changing some habits.

When the upper back and shoulders are kept strong and supple, they prevent aches and pains from rounding and drooping. Fully developed, as in the case of weight lifters, dancers, or gymnasts, they look like sensual, sculptured, convoluted mounds and crevices coiling along the upper back and separated by one deep, clean-cut line that sharply divides the two halves of the back down the center. Most of us, however, would be satisfied with enough development to simply straighten ourselves out of a slouch.

In this chapter, the exercises are designed to help keep your shoulders straight, to expand your chest, and to strengthen your upper back. Movements that carry the arms overhead or backward help to strengthen the shoulders and to stretch the chest muscles. Movements that hold the shoulders and head back also help correct a stooped posture.

Naturally, any of the exercises in this chapter should be reinforced by some daily habits that help you broaden and widen your shoulders, expand and unfold your upper body, and flower open to the world!

Your Naked Neck

Imagine a 10-pound pumpkin delicately balancing atop a single mattress spring, and you can better appreciate the work of your neck. Your head is a heavy segment perched atop seven rather small, pliable neck vertebrae. It's a topheavy package that is kept from toppling by neck muscles controlling the head's every position. Muscles in the back of your neck are especially responsible for the balancing act; by contracting when the head moves, they keep the head stabilized. When the neck muscles become flaccid from lack of exercise, gravity, which exerts a constant nagging pull on the heavy head, begins to win the tug-of-war over your yielding neck muscles.

The more physically monotonous occupations of modern man and woman have the head hanging from the neck as it pores over desk work. By allowing our head to dribble down (for whatever reason) we are instigating an avalanche of the upper body, beginning with the hanging head, to the stooped shoulders, to the caving chest. Like dominoes, we weaken all the muscles along the way that were meant to keep the parts erect.

Eventually, those feeble neck muscles are subjected to great strain in their attempts to keep the habitually hanging head in balance. Fatigued beyond their endurance, these poor muscles protest by pulsating a pain in the neck, and passing it on to the shoulders. We suffer from a headache, a stiff neck, or a stab between the shoulder blades. By keeping the neck flexible the pain and tension in these areas can be relieved.

The naked neck is one area of your body that is constantly exposed to public viewing. Elongated, toned neck muscles reveal a slender, streamlined contour. Lethargic, foreshortened neck muscles bare layers of chin rolls, one thick puff that protrudes in front from chin to collarbone, or one dowager's hump that protrudes in the back.

Think of your neck as an area of personal expressiveness. A supple, graceful, long neck creates the illusion of confidently opening out to the world. A rigid neck creates the illusion of tension and of constricted self-expression—a turtle receding into its shell.

The actual contour of the neck varies with age. Eventually the skin will lose its resilience and some fatty deposits will appear under the chin. Cosmetic surgery aside, usually a combination of exercise and a change in the habitual way of holding your head can carve your neck into more streamlined proportions.

Isometric-resistive-type exercises develop strength in the neck. Use your hands, or any resistive force, to press against a part of your head, then try to push your head against the pressure of your hands (or the force) for 8 counts

before relaxing. Neck-stretches are provided in this chapter and permeate other chapters. While you exercise your neck, keep in mind that your movements should be smooth and fluid, not jerky.

The very best neck exercise is constant, daily postural reinforcement. If you gently tuck in your chin and lift it slightly, instead of jutting it forward and down, then the curve in the back of your neck can straighten to balance your head. Imagine clusters of balloons lightly attached to your ears by long strings. As the balloons softly raise in the breeze, the spaces between the neck vertebrae begin to expand and your neck gently elongates up through your crown, which should float on top!

The Technique: Chest-Arm Builders

Isometric Push-ups

These push-ups are designed to firm the arm, chest, and shoulder muscles.

Position: Lie on your stomach with legs together, toes curled under, and palms flat on the floor next to the chest. Tighten every muscle, making the body flat and rigid like a board.

Beginners: Press the hands firmly into the floor as you lift the upper torso a few inches; hold for 2 counts. Then lift it a few more inches and hold for 2 counts.

Now straighten the elbows as you push up to your knees. Keep the back flat. Stop one-third of

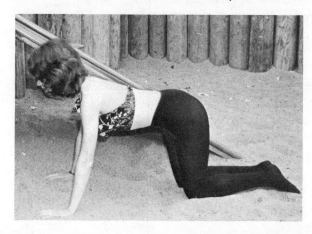

the way down and hold. Stop again at the two-thirds mark before touching the floor. Repeat these half-push-ups 4 or more times in a row. Don't be discouraged if once is your limit. When your arms feel strong enough, try the intermediate version.

Intermediates: Follow the beginner half-push-up to the knees. From there, straighten your legs and elbows so that just the toes and hands are on the floor. Flatten out your body.

Push down by bending the elbows, lowering one-third of the way. Stop and hold for 2 counts. Lower two-thirds of the way; stop and hold for 2 counts. Now touch the floor, chest first. Repeat the half-push-up/full-push-down sequence at least twice, more if possible.

Advanced: Push up with straight legs. Legs and chest lift simultaneously—no cheating by lifting the head and chest first. Lower to the floor the

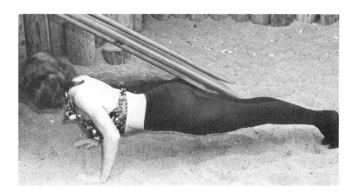

same way. Try several without pausing. Remember to make 2 stops on the ascent and 2 on the descent.

Body Awareness: To make your body stiffer and stronger, pull the stomach in and squeeze the buttocks together, keeping it level with your back. Do you feel strength emanating from the arm, shoulder, and chest muscles?

Kneeling Push-ups

Push-ups are an excellent way to build strength into weak chest and arm muscles. Here's a variation that everyone can try, the degree of difficulty depending mainly on where you place your hands.

Position: Get down on all fours, with your hands placed shoulder-width apart. Flatten your back so it is parallel to the floor, draw your stomach in, and straighten your elbows.

Beginners: Bend your elbows out as you lower your chest to the floor in 2 counts. Hold for 2 counts, then press your hands hard on the floor to straighten your elbows again as you lift your chest. The idea is to touch only your chest to the floor. You're cheating if you sit back when your elbows bend. Repeat 10–20 times, or as long as stamina permits. Try not to rush your counts; push down and up very slowly.

Intermediates: Alter the position so your hands are wide apart and your lower legs are bent up off the floor. Now you are supported by your hands and knees only, with most of your weight on the hands. In this position, follow the beginner exercise.

Advanced: Place your hands close together under your chest and bend your lower legs up off the floor. Follow the beginner version in this position, trying to touch your nose to the floor.

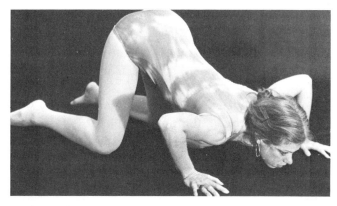

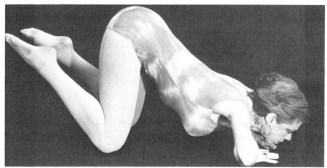

Body Awareness: It's tempting to "sit" back when you lower your chest to the floor, but you won't obtain the full strength value from the exercise. Instead, try to lean slightly forward when you push down. Are you feeling your chest, forearms, upper arms, and shoulders building strength? You might also feel a back stretch.

Frog Push-ups

Here's a super toner for weak arm, chest, and shoulder muscles.

Position: Squat down with the feet together and heels up. Place your hands flat on the floor alongside the knees, with the fingers facing outward.

Beginners: Keeping your elbows straight, lean forward slowly for 4 counts until your knees come to about an inch from the floor. Hold the lean for 4 counts, then rock back on 4. Repeat twice more without pausing. Relax, then try the set again.

Intermediates: Perform the beginner exercise as above, but bend your elbows as you lean forward on 4 counts. Hold the lean for 4 with bent elbows. Return to center and straighten the elbows. Repeat twice more without pausing. Relax, then try the set again.

Advanced: Straighten up your legs and lift your heels so your weight is forward onto your hands. Turn the hands so the fingers face straight ahead. Now bend the elbows as you lower your upper torso on 4 slow counts until your nose is almost touching the floor. Hold for 4 (keep smiling) then straighten the elbows on 4. Repeat twice (or more) without pausing. Relax, then repeat for as long as stamina permits.

Body Awareness: For maximum benefit, try not to rush your counts, and don't let the shoulders hunch up. You should be feeling muscles in the arms, chest, and shoulders building strength! In the advanced version, you'll also feel a surprise stretch along the back and legs.

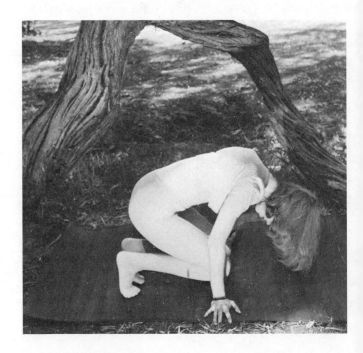

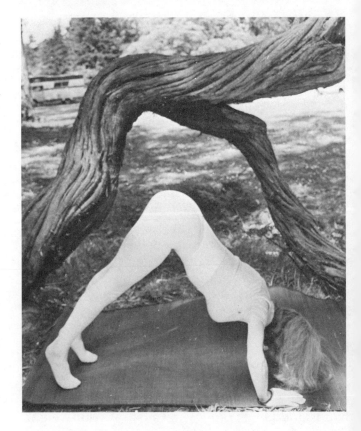

Sideways Push-ups

Position: Lie on your right side and support your upper body on your extended right arm, with the left hand behind your head.

Beginners: In one count, thrust your hips off the floor so you're supported diagonally on just the outer edge of your right foot and your right hand. On the second count, lower your hips to just a few inches from the floor. Alternate lowering and raising your hips sideways for 4–8 counts, keeping the supporting arm straight. Shake out your wrist, change sides, and repeat. Try the set 2–4 more times.

Intermediates: Follow the beginner version. Each time you lower your hip, let it touch the floor before you thrust it up again.

Advanced: Raise your hip off the floor. Now stay up as you kick your free leg up and down 8 times. Kick as high as you can, keeping the knee straight and the toes pointed. Change sides and repeat. Try the set again.

Body Awareness: Don't be discouraged if at first you can't support your body weight on one hand and foot. With consistent practice you will develop enough strength in the wrists, forearms, and upper arms to accomplish the exercise!

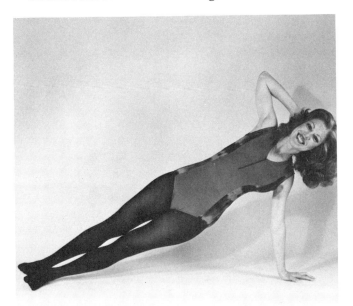
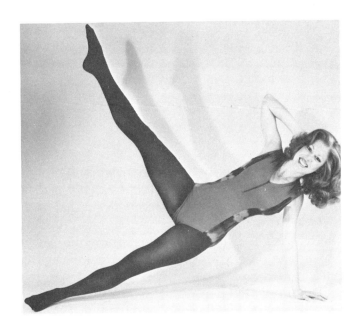

The Pusher

Build up the chest muscles as you strengthen your arms and shoulders.

Position: Stand arm's distance from a wall, or support, with legs together and straight. Squeeze your buttocks and shrink your stomach.

Beginners: Place your hands, turned inward, against a wall or support at chest level. Fingers are turned in a few inches apart. Elbows are straight. Take 4 counts to lean forward as you bend the elbows. Keep your back straight. Just before your nose touches the support, stop and hold for 4 counts. Straighten on 4. Repeat without pausing 2–4 times. Relax, then repeat the set once more or as stamina permits.

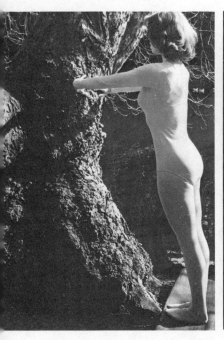
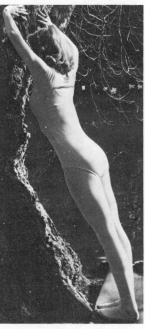

Intermediates: Follow the beginner exercise with your hands raised to shoulder level against the support. Increase the hold to 8 counts. Try the set 2–4 times without pausing. Repeat if stamina permits.

Advanced: Raise your hands as high against the support as is possible, still keeping the palms flat, the fingers facing in, and the elbows straight. Now follow the intermediate exercise.

Body Awareness: As you lean forward, you should be contracting your buttocks together and maintaining a straight back. Don't look down. Are you feeling the chest, arms, and shoulders building strength? You might also feel the buttock muscles toning and the calf muscles stretching.

Pinwheels

Give yourself a whirl—here's an invigorating toner for the chest, arms, and shoulders. It's also a great warm-up exercise to stimulate circulation.

Position: Stand with your feet about shoulder-width apart. Lengthen your spine, draw your stomach in, and press your shoulders down and slightly back.

Beginners: In 4 peppy counts: Swing your right arm sideways to shoulder level, now swing it across your body (keeping the elbow straight), swing it sideways and whirl it all the way around twice, describing 2 complete circles in front of your body. Repeat. Without pausing, reverse the direction of the arm swings for 2 sets: Start with the arm across your body, then swing it out to the side, then whirl it twice. Change arms for 4 sets. Relax, then repeat the entire sequence 4 times or until the arms feel tired.

Intermediates and Advanced: Follow the beginner exercise, using both arms simultaneously. Press up onto the balls of your feet when you: swing both arms *out to* the sides, swing them across your body crisscross style, and start to whirl them around. Repeat the set 4 times, then immediately reverse the direction of the arms for 4 sets (begin with the arms crisscrossed in front of you). Relax, then repeat the entire exercise sequence once or twice more.

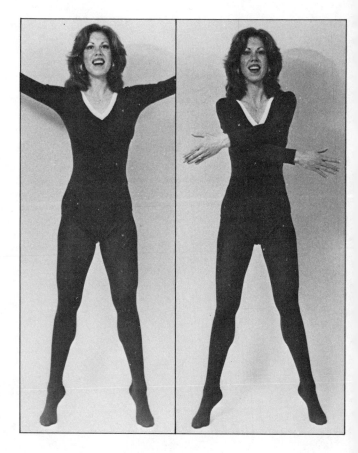

Body Awareness: While your arms are whirling out, across, or around in a continuous flow, try not to bend your elbows. You may hear a crackling sound in the shoulder bones as they loosen.

Snap-backs

Snap out of a slouch! If your back, shoulders, and chest are stiff from slouching, this exercise will help to loosen and straighten them.

Position: Sit with your knees bent up just enough so your feet are flat on the floor. The hands are on the floor next to your hips, and your back is very straight.

Beginners: Sit flush up against a wall in the above position. Imagine that your hips, back, shoulders, and neck are melting into the wall. Raise one arm straight up past the ear and try to press your arm to the wall. If your shoulders and upper back are stiff, don't expect to be able to touch the wall behind you with a straight elbow. Let the elbow bend as much as is necessary.

Hold the arm to the wall for 8–12 slow counts, then change arms for 8–12 counts. Now try to press and hold both arms overhead against the wall for 12 counts. Repeat the set 4 times in succession, striving to keep the arms as straight as possible.

Intermediates: Assume the same position as the beginners', without using the wall for support. Straighten one arm overhead so it passes close to the ear, then snap it backward 8 times, keeping the elbow straight. While the arm snaps back, let your chest pulsate forward slightly. Change arms for 8, then snap both arms back for 12 counts while the chest pulsates forward. Repeat the set 4 times in succession. You're cheating if you let your back round.

Advanced: Follow the intermediate version, sitting with your knees close to your chest and heels as close to your bottom as possible.

Body Awareness: The closer your arms are to the ears and the straighter the elbows, the harder this exercise is. It may look deceptively easy to perform, but it is quite a challenge at any level. Daily practice will help to straighten your back and shoulders.

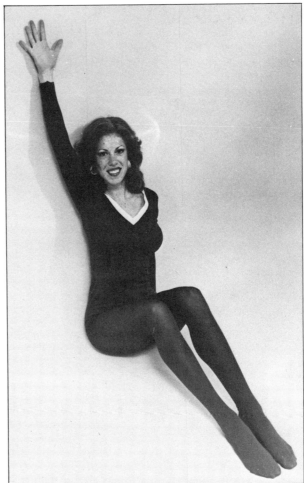

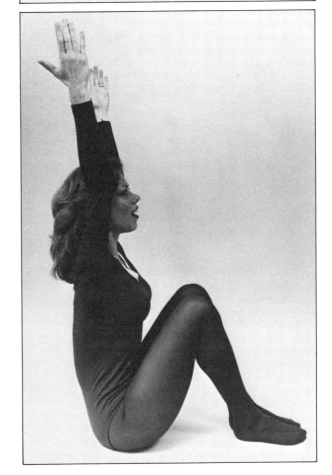

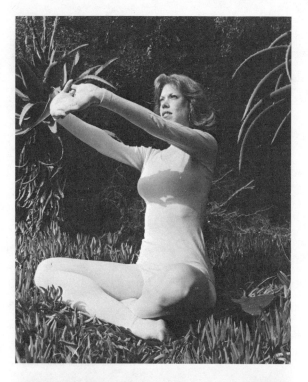

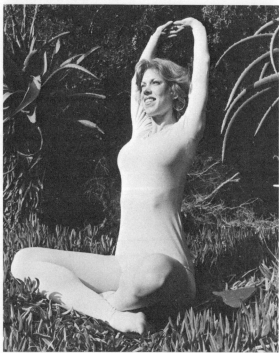

The Palms Stretch

Position: Sit squarely on your buttocks, with the feet crossed at your ankles. Lace your fingers, then stretch your arms forward at shoulder level, with the palms turned outward.

Beginners: Sit flush against a wall or other back support. Raise your arms straight overhead (or higher if you can) in 2 counts. As the arms raise up, press your shoulders *down* and draw them back. Lower the arms to shoulder level in 2 counts. When you lower the arms, feel as though you were pushing against a resistance. Continue raising and lowering slowly 8–16 times in a row. Relax the arms a moment, then repeat the set.

Intermediates and Advanced: Follow the beginner version without using a back support. Try to raise your arms higher to just in front of your ears.

Now raise your arms overhead behind your ears. Keeping your fingers laced, bounce the arms in back of the ears 8 times. Don't let your head poke forward—keep it perched firmly on your neck! Lower the arms on 4, then raise them overhead again and repeat the bounces. Try a third set if stamina permits.

Body Awareness: You're cheating if your elbows are bent even a fraction, or if your shoulders and back start to round. Try to keep your back flat and straight. Are you feeling the arm and shoulder muscles building strength as the chest muscles are being stretched?

The Rope Stretch

Here's an exercise that rescues you from slumped posture. With the help of a rope or stick, you can straighten your shoulders and expand your chest to its maximum.

Position: Sit on the floor with your legs crossed, "Indian style." Grasp a rope (or long towel, stick, etc.) with your hands placed a little farther than shoulder-width apart. Straighten your spine and contract your stomach.

Beginners: Keeping your elbows absolutely straight, stretch your arms forward and up, bringing the rope overhead in 4 slow counts. While you hold the rope overhead, bounce-pulsate your arms slightly behind your ears for 8 counts. Now lower the arms and rest for a moment. Repeat 4–8 times, never letting your elbows bend.

Intermediates: After you bounce-pulsate the arms 8 times, continue to stretch the rope past your ears and all the way back behind you. When you reach your middle back, stop and hold the stretch for 4 counts. Then slowly raise the rope up, overhead, and down in front. Repeat the exercise 6–8 times without pausing.

Advanced: Follow the intermediate exercise with your hands placed shoulder-width apart, or closer if possible.

Body Awareness: The closer your hands are, the more difficult this exercise becomes. You'll find the stretch more effective if you perform the exercise slowly; don't rush your counts. It's outright cheating if you poke your head forward, if you lean forward, or if you bend your elbows!

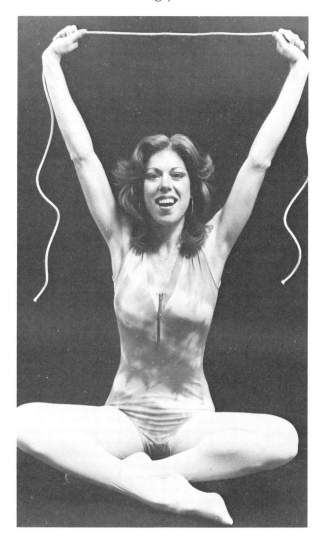
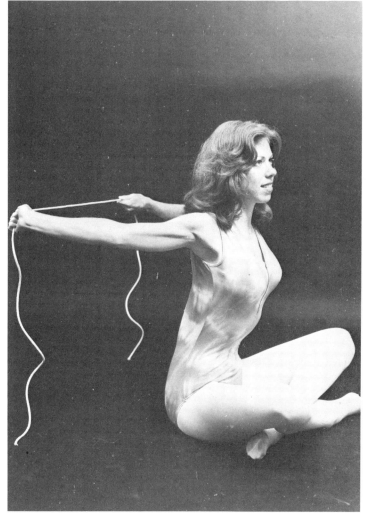

Flour Power

Flabby arms are especially disturbing when you're all dressed up in your sleeveless finery, and the rest of you looks terrific except for the loose sacks exposed and flopping about from your shoulders. The flaccid flesh is partly due to unused arm muscles, so you'll need to start using your upper arms every day. Gradually you'll be placing more stress on the muscles and they will develop more strength.

Start with two sacks of all-purpose flour (or sugar) weighing 5 pounds each. Don't cook with them. Instead, lie on the floor on your back with your knees up and stomach drawn in so that your lower back touches the floor. Hold a sack in each hand and extend your arms straight up to the ceiling. In 4 slow counts, lower your arms as you slant them slightly backward. Try to lower them as close to the floor as possible, then immediately raise them, using 4 slow counts. Don't bend your elbows and don't rush your counts. Repeat that exercise *slowly* as many times as you can without pausing. Strive for 10 in a row. Relax for a few seconds, then repeat another set.

If you'd like more of an arm-*and*-chest strengthener, try this variation: In 4 counts, lower your arms sideways to the floor (slant them back slightly

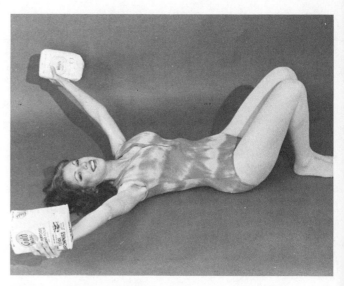

as in the photo). Raise them straight up on 4. Repeat the sequence—up, side, up, back—10 times without pausing. Relax, then repeat another set of 10.

Body Awareness: If your arms and chest muscles are really weak, you may not be able to accomplish a full set of 10 lifts. Once you build strength in the muscles and 2 or 3 sets of 10 lifts feel too easy for you, then increase the weights by 2–3 pounds. Be sure the bags are sealed tight!

Dumbbell Hints

Serious weight workouts are now incorporated into the training sessions of most professional athletes (both men and women) as an effective way to increase strength, power, and stamina. If you want to supplement your own regular sports or fitness program, you can add a few exercises using weights. As in any fitness program, you'll want to be absolutely sure that your body is warmed up thoroughly before you start lifting weights. Entering any kind of physical training without a warm-up period first is an invitation to injury. Give yourself at least 15–20 minutes of cardiovascular and flexibility exercises before you tackle weights, and your body should be prepared for the more demanding resistance workout.

In the case of any weight-lifting exercise, be very sure that you completely extend your arm

with the weight. If you stop before your arm completely straightens, you will not develop to your full strength potential. If you allow your back to sway while you're lifting weights, as in the second photo, you can easily rupture the lower-back vertebrae and set yourself up for pain you hadn't planned on. When possible, weight-lift in front of a mirror so you can correct your posture and avoid back injury.

When you're confined to a small area, exercising with dumbbells can be one effective way to tone up. There are several different dumbbell exercises that will help strengthen the chest muscles, tone the arms (especially those loose sacks of flesh in the back of the arms), and strengthen the biceps and forearms.

Here's one simple exercise. Choose a pair of

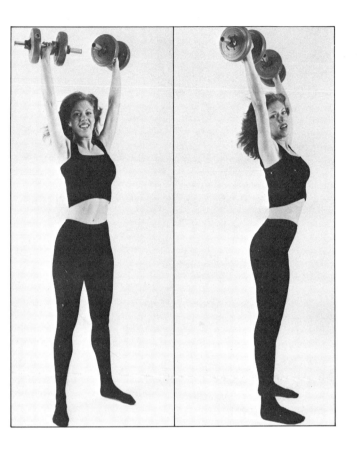

dumbbells that aren't so heavy that you cannot complete the proper number of sets and repetitions. A suggested starting weight for women might be a pair that weighs 3–5 pounds each. Stand with your feet a little more than shoulder-width apart and hold a dumbbell in each hand at shoulder level with elbows close to your sides. Press one dumbbell overhead (straighten the arm completely) as you inhale. Exhale when you lower it to shoulder height, then raise the other hand overhead. Continue alternating arms 20 times (10 each arm). After a few weeks gradually add more arm movement, until you're doing 15 repetitions per arm. Then add more weight (3–5 lbs) to each dumbbell and begin again with 10 repetitions. You can try pressing both dumbbells overhead simultaneously for your second set. If it's strength you want, you'll need to increase the resistance gradually as your muscles adjust to a certain load. If you desire stamina, then increase the number of repetitions or sets without increasing the resistance.

The Technique: Neck-Shoulder Builders

The Neck Arch

A little serious necking: Develop a long, slender neck by arching and stretching it.

Position: Lie on your back with the stomach contracted, feet together, and hands at your sides.

Beginners: In 4 counts, arch the back of your neck up off the floor so the top of your head (or as close to the top as possible) is touching the floor and you are gazing backward. Hold the neck arch as you open and close your mouth 4 times as if you were chewing. Now roll the neck down so it is flat on the floor with your chin tucked in (4 counts). Repeat the sequence 4–6 times or until the neck feels well stretched.

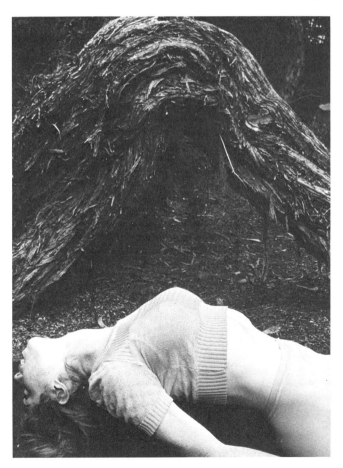

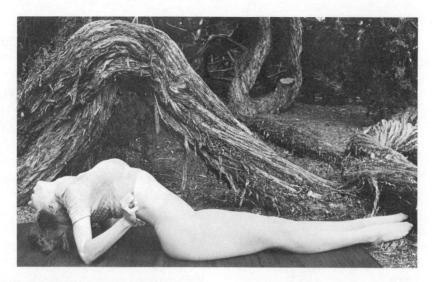

Intermediates: Follow the beginner version, but dig your elbows into the floor at your sides when you arch your neck up. You should be arching farther back so the forehead is closer to the floor behind you.

Advanced: Dig your elbows into the floor and arch up to the top of your head. Now lift your head one inch off the floor and hold as you chew 4 times (open and close your mouth). Roll the neck down again until it is flat on the floor. Repeat 4 times or until the neck feels tired.

Body Awareness: As you arch the neck, keep your shoulders down and back; don't let them hunch up toward your ears. Think about pressing your stomach and shoulders into the floor when the neck is flattening. Do you feel both the front and back neck muscles stretching?

Neck Rolls

To relieve neck and upper-back tension as you slenderize the neck muscles.

Position: Stand or sit with your back elongated and the chest lifted. Draw the stomach muscles in gently.

Drops: Drop your head forward from the base of the neck without rounding the shoulders. Now plop it over to the right side (right ear toward the shoulder). Then dangle it back with your mouth closed to feel the chin and neck muscles stretch. End with the head dropped to the left. Sustain each drop for 2 counts. Repeat, then reverse direction of the drops, starting counterclockwise. Repeat.

Circles: Continue the above exercise by circling the head around very slowly and smoothly clockwise. Make 2–4 generous circles, then reverse direction for 2–4 more. Feel deeply relaxed as the head slowly circles and the neck muscles stretch.

Body Awareness: Keep the shoulders relaxed but immobile; you are isolating movement in the neck and head only. If you feel dizzy, shake your head from side to side a few quick times. Do you feel the neck muscles stretching as you become more relaxed?

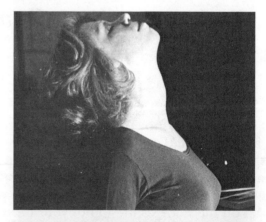

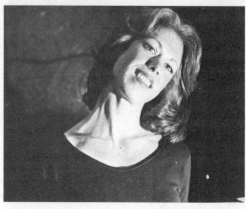

The Gobbler

Toning a turkey neck: A little effective gobbling can combat a double chin and sagging neck muscles. While you're still young, take a few minutes every day and try this easy toner that helps prevent your chin from dropping down into your neck.

Position: Sit up very straight with your knees bent, feet flat on the floor and palms on the floor right behind your hips.

Start: Drop your head forward from the base of your neck and aim the chin to your chest. In 4 counts, lift your chin up so that it points to the ceiling. Now press your hands on the floor, push your chest forward, and drop the head farther back so that you feel a superstretch along the neck. Hold it there for 4 slow counts as you draw your shoulders down and back.

With your head dangling backward, open and close your mouth four times, as if you were chewing or gobbling. Now tilt your head slightly to one side and chew 4 times, then tilt it to the other side and chew 4 times.

Lower your chin to chest, then repeat the entire exercise 2–4 more times.

Body Awareness: This exercise reads a lot easier than it really is! If you're doing it correctly, you'll feel a great stretch all along the neck and chin. Be careful not to overpull the muscles by arching *too* far.

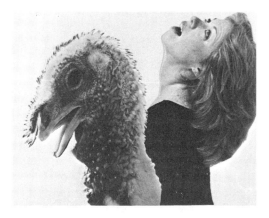

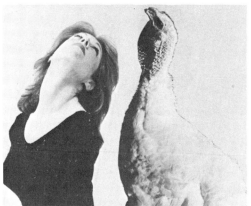

Shoulder Rolls

A tension reliever for stiff neck and shoulder muscles.

Position: Sit or stand with your back lengthened.

Single Rolls: 1. Roll just the right shoulder forward without moving the left one. 2. Now lift the right shoulder up toward your ear. 3. Shift it back. 4. Press it down and center. Use 4 slow counts, pausing briefly to hold the shoulder in each of the 4 directions. Repeat the set of 4 (with pauses) twice. Then reverse direction (beginning back) for 3 sets. Now roll the shoulder smoothly around, as above, without a pause. Try the smooth rolls twice in each direction, then change shoulders and repeat the above sequence with the left.

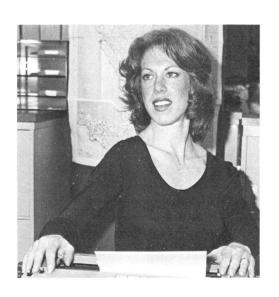

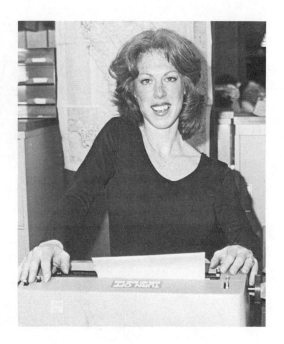

Both Shoulders: Perform the above set, rolling both shoulders simultaneously. You may want to repeat the entire exercise twice more, beginning with the single rolls.

Body Awareness: Since this is a shoulder-isolation movement, try not to use the neck muscles. Keep the head very still. Also, try not to move the left shoulder when the right is working, and vice versa. If you keep the rolls smooth and slow, you will feel a soothing, relaxing effect begin to replace any strains felt in the upper-back region.

Racket Stretch

Tennis is wonderful exercise *if* you can find a court! Unfortunately, too often this popular sport turns into a game of waiting around for a court or a space at the backboard, especially on weekends. Next time you're keeping the bench warm watching the other players, try this simple warm-up stretch. This exercise will loosen the arm, chest, and shoulder muscles, allowing you a fuller, freer swing when you serve and return the ball.

Grasp the racket at both ends and straighten your arms in front of you. Now sit up very straight and raise the racket overhead. Keep pulling the racket backward until you've reached your stretch limit, without letting your elbows bend or your head poke forward. Count to 8, then lower your arms.

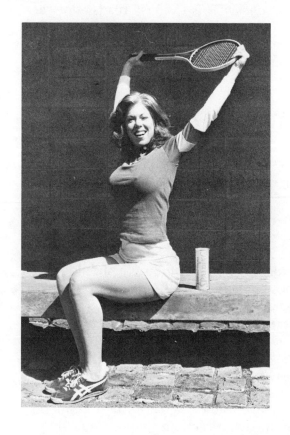

The second time you do the exercise, bring your racket up and overhead as far back as you can. Instead of holding for 8, bounce your arms backward (past your ears) 8 times, then lower them.

Repeat this stretch until you feel your back, arms, and shoulders loosening.

Body Awareness: You're cheating if you let your shoulders round, your head poke forward, or your elbows bend!

Secret Chest Exercises

Here are a few hints to help you concentrate on your chest muscles. These may seem innocent enough, but they will help to give you a real lift during the day!

- Using heavy cookware daily instead of the lightweight kind helps to build up your arm and chest muscles.
- If you leave the market with only one or two bundles, discard the cart and carry the bundles close to your chest.
- While sitting at a desk, try pressing your fists hard against the desk top and try to lift your body up off the seat without leaning forward (elbows close to your sides).
- Whenever you move your arms, try to begin the movement from the shoulder joint, not the elbow.
- When you squeeze water from a washcloth or sponge, wring it until you feel the exertion in your arms and wrists.
- When you pass under a door frame, occasionally press against the sides with your hands. Press with all your might for 6 counts, keeping the shoulder tips down, then pass on through.
- Vacuuming, lifting, shoveling, mowing the lawn, and throwing all help to develop your chest and arms.

Shoulder-Neck Hints

- Be in the habit of drawing the shoulders gently back and level when you sit, stand, walk—wherever you are, whatever you're doing.
- When you carry any weighty object, don't let the shoulder slump on that side. Keep it level. Try not to carry a purse, suitcase, camera (or any strapped object) over one shoulder only, or with one hand only. Give the other side equal carrying time!
- Be sure your table or desk isn't too high, or you'll cause the shoulders to bunch up and the neck to shorten, inducing strain in those muscles. You should be able to place your forearms on your desk without your shoulders lifting up. Don't hesitate to take short exercise breaks during work time to roll and stretch the neck and shoulders.
- While you pore over your work, try not to let your head dangle. Instead, hold it up and lean over from your hips. If your desk is too low, then your head and shoulders will tend to drop.
- Avoid chairs with high backs that cause your head to poke forward.
- If you read in bed, don't pile pillows under your neck so your chin is pressing onto your chest. Instead, sit up flush against a backrest.
- Try to sleep without a pillow, or use just a thin type. Avoid the stuffed, spongy pillows that prop your neck out of alignment.
- Try washing your hair in the shower with your back to the water so your neck stretches backward during the rinse.
- When you glance up to look overhead, don't just raise your eyes. Keep your back straight and use your neck muscles to exaggerate the head-tilt way back, so you feel a stretch under your chin.
- When you turn to look over your shoulder, exaggerate the twist so you really feel the sides of your neck stretch.

CHAPTER SIX:

HOW TO HAVE SHAPELY LOWER LEGS

Two exposed slender shafts—each with a shapely, carved curve in the back that tapers down to a slim indentation at the ankle—are provocative! Some people are born with gorgeous legs, but most of us have to work for them, else we lose all definition in the shafts, and may have a normal body perched on two thick trunks.

The lower legs, that part between the feet and thighs, are the supportive trunks that bear the stressful weight of the body from above and transmit it to the roots below. When they are weak and underdeveloped, they lack a shapely contour. But even worse, weak leg muscles can grow misshapen, making them vulnerable to cramps and injury. The long lower-leg bone connects to the knee joint above and the foot below. Since both the knees and feet are vulnerable to stress and injury, both acting as shock absorbers when weight is placed on them, they depend upon the shin, calf, and thigh muscles to be strong and to help keep them stable.

Shapely lower legs should walk with a light, buoyant, graceful gait. The springy lightness in our walk depends on the condition of our feet, the strength and flexibility of the muscles surrounding the ankle joint and heel cord, and on the arches and toes themselves.

When we're running, jumping, or suspended in balance, the power for the feet to perform comes from the calf muscles. The heel cord or Achilles tendon, the strongest tendon in our body, gives the bend, spring, and leap ability to our feet. Buoyant, free motion starts from elastic calf muscles and Achilles tendons, both sets allowing the foot to rotate and the toes to push off for real action. Our feet are the springboards for all our locomotion and transfer of the body's weight. While the feet are active, the supporting arches act like cushions absorbing shock. If they are stiff, weak, or misaligned, then our walk is heavy and slothful.

As the basic support and foundation on which the rest of our body balances, those little feet contain no less than one-quarter of all the bones in the body! Strong, supple foot muscles give the body a firm foundation for its support. Any weakness or stiffness in the toes, arches, or ankles will send signals of instability throughout your entire body, causing the parts to tumble into disarray. Just like muscles in the rest of the body, unused foot muscles grow weak and stiff.

An estimated 80 percent of the adult population suffers from some kind of foot misery. In our daily civilized life, the feet are encased in (usually) uncomfortable shoes that pound on hard pavement. The poor foot muscles become mummified in their very encasements. The little toes become brittle from insufficient use and, depending on the shoes, may grow crooked or bent. The heel cord shortens and stiffens, and the arches weaken, if the heels are too high. Very high heels throw the body's weight forward onto the balls of the feet, causing the arches to weaken and the toes to cramp. If the heels are constantly elevated in platform or high-heeled shoes, the tendons and calf muscles shorten and become inelastic. Eventually they grow stiff, and we suffer from low-back pain or calf cramps (charley horses).

Another common ailment is weak or fallen arches, caused by habitually bearing the body's weight on the inner borders of the feet. When the arches roll in to accept the weight, the ankles, knees, and thighs also rotate in knock-knee style. Long hours of standing can make the arches sag and weaken. Obesity also puts chronic excessive pressure on the foot muscles, eventually causing the decline and fall of the supportive arches.

In daily strolling, foot misalignments create strains and cramps in your feet and lower legs; in sports, misalignments are often the instigator of serious injuries. With increasing age and disuse, the foot muscles and joints eventually cramp our walking style. Tired, burning, swollen feet; sprained ankles; fatigue, slumped posture; lower leg pains—all stem from weak, flat, or misaligned feet and uncomfortable shoes. Nothing makes you ache all over like a pair of aching feet! In most cases cramps are preventable just by wearing low-heeled shoes more often, by exercising your leg and foot muscles, and by learning to use your feet correctly.

Through developing the foot muscles, they can be made more supple and supportive. You'll also want to keep the calf and shin muscles stretched to avoid leg cramps. When the lower legs are kept strong, they can better absorb shock and stabilize the ankles to keep them from flopping and twisting. Face it: a proud, light saunter is simply an impossible achievement on a set of feeble feet. By learning to develop all parts of our roots, we allow the branches above to be better balanced and supported.

The Technique

Adult's Play: Jumping Rope

Déjà vu? Remember skipping rope during recess and never feeling winded? Well, guess which childhood game is having a revival. Fair warning: Jumping rope is no mere child's play! It is excellent cardiovascular exercise for adults and kids which requires consistent practice to endure for more than a few minutes. If your heart and lungs are out of condition, you can expect to become breathless in one minute flat. Jumping rope is one of the best ways to keep the feet, calves, thighs, and heart muscle strong. It also challenges your coordination.

Don't be discouraged at your first attempt if you've never jumped rope before (or haven't done it in years). It is more demanding staminawise than jogging; and it will take practice to coordinate the rope so that it doesn't get all tangled between your feet.

The Rope: Unwaxed clothesline or number-10 sash cord make fine jump ropes. Stand in the middle of the loop and cut the ends so they come to just below your armpits.

Beginner's skip-rope (jump twice for every turn of the rope): Once over the rope lightly, then a smaller bounce follows while the rope raises overhead. Try to keep your jumps continuous and rhythmic for at least 1 minute, then work up to 5 minutes nonstop. For stamina, equate 1 minute of this double-bounce style to 2 minutes of jogging. Subtract the seconds it takes you to pick up the rope every time it drops! (See Chapter Eight for cardiovascular benefits.)

Intermediates' Jump-Rope (one bounce to each turn of the rope): You're moving faster, so equate 1 minute of this single-bounce style to 3 minutes of jogging. Make your goal 5 minutes of single bouncing without stopping.

Advanced: Try to perform fancy rope-crosses while you turn the rope forward and backward overhead. Then try hopping, running, kicking, etc., while the rope turns. Try all sorts of fancy steps while you jump nonstop for at least 5 minutes.

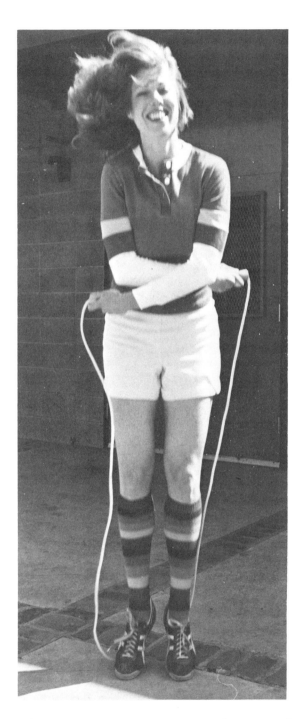

Body Awareness: Beginning students tend to jump too high or turn the rope with their arms held too far out to the sides. Keep your jumps very small and your arm movements down to a minimum. Actually, the hands do most of the turning, not the arms. It was fun and exercise back then, and you'll rediscover the same now!

Jumper Heel-ups

If you're planning to involve yourself in summer sports, you'll want to stand up to the stress placed upon your feet. This jumping exercise will help strengthen your feet and ankles in preparation for any physical demands, and help to increase cardiovascular stamina.

Position: Stand with good posture: stomach drawn in, back lengthened, shoulders relaxed, and head up. Contract your buttocks and tuck them in slightly. Open your arms to the sides. Your feet are positioned so that heels are together and toes are apart.

Beginners: Touch a wall or support. Now bend your knees so that they open wide over the toes. Bend them as low as you can in 4 counts, keeping your heels on the floor. While the knees are bent, lift just your heels high off the floor in 4 counts. Keep the heels up as you straighten the legs in 4 more counts. Now hold for 4, then lower the heels to the floor. Repeat the set at least 6 times without pausing.

Intermediates: Follow the beginner exercise without holding onto a support.

Advanced: Bend your knees wide over your toes in 4 counts. Now jump up high in the air and straighten both legs and point the toes. As you land from the jump, bend your knees and land on the balls of your feet first, then lower your heels. Straighten your legs in 2 counts. Continue the exercise 8 times without a pause. Relax, then repeat for 8 more.

Body Awareness: If you lose your balance, recheck the posture principles above. To build strength in your feet and ankles, remember to lift those heels high enough off the floor so that you are on your toes. Your weight should be centered over the big toes. Feel the calves, ankles, and toes building strength?

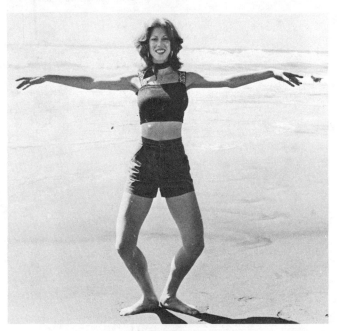

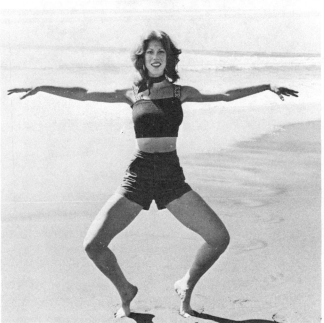

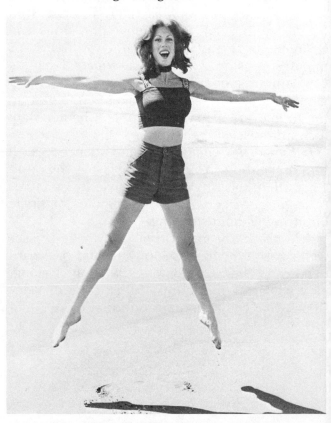

Jumping-Jack Alternatives

No exercise program is effective unless you begin with a hearty warm-up that stimulates the cardio-vascular system, getting the blood circulating throughout your entire body. Traditionally, "jumping jacks"—that old, familiar calisthenic-style exercise—was used to warm up a group of not-so-willing exercise recruits. But these days there are more creative, enjoyable ways to warm up. Some people use jogging or jumping rope as an excellent warm-up for their exercise session. Here are a few jumping alternatives guaranteed to keep your corpuscles moving!

Heel Clicks: You've seen these in Gene Kelly musicals. Spread your arms sideways and take 3 small running steps, starting with the right foot. On the 4th count, kick the left foot out to the side and immediately lift the right foot so that the right heel "clicks" against the left heel. The "clicks" happen on the 4th beat. Without pausing, take 3 running steps with your left foot, and on the 4th count kick the right foot sideways, then lift the left heel up to the right one. Continue this way, alternating feet, 10–16 times. Each time strive for a higher kick to the side, so that you're jumping each time you click heels. Now try taking only 1 step, then click heels, alternating side to side, 8–16 times.

Hops: Spread your arms sideways and place your right toes behind your left knee. Jump 4 times on the left foot, then immediately switch sides (left toes behind the right knee) for 4 counts, then jump 4 times with feet together. Whenever you jump, you bend the knees first in preparation, and land on the balls of the feet first. For the second set, try to jump higher. For the third set, your jumps should have more elevation and you'll become airborne! Finally, for the last set, you'll be leaping high 8 times on each foot and 8 times with feet together. There's no pause between sets!

Leaping Frog (not for people with knee problems): Jump high on both feet and land in a squat position. Repeat several times.

Bird Jumps: Jump up and touch the bottoms of your feet together under you. Jump a second time, spread legs apart, and try to touch your toes while the legs are in mid-air (advanced). Repeat, alternating the footwork (feet together, then legs apart) for as long as stamina permits.

With a little imagination I'm sure you can de-

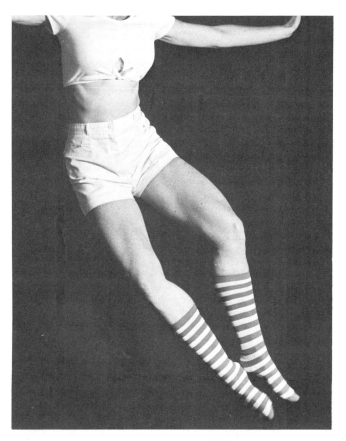

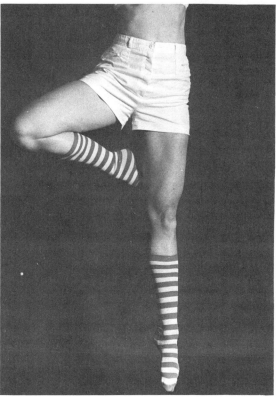

vise your own jump routines. If you're still stuck on jumping jacks, then occasionally add a variation: do a half or full turn every third or fourth time you jump.

Heel-ups

Here's an exercise that builds strength into weak feet, ankles, and flabby thighs while it develops better balance.

Position: Stand with your feet wide apart and turned out a bit so the toes face east and west. Elongate your spine, shrink your stomach, and straighten your knees. Think tall.

Beginners: Touch a wall for support. In 4 slow counts, bend your knees directly over your toes without leaning forward. Keep your buttocks tucked under you (don't let them protrude when you bend). Hold the bent position for 8 slow counts, with the knees bent low and wide so they're aligned over your toes. Now lift just your heels high off the floor and hold for 8 counts. By now you'll want to slowly straighten your knees completely. Stiffen the knees and ankles as you balance on your toes for 8 counts, then lower the heels to the floor with the knees kept straight.

Repeat the entire exercise without pausing 6–8 times, or as long as stamina permits.

Intermediates: Follow the beginner exercise without touching the wall. Instead, stretch your arms out to the sides to help you balance.

Advanced: Perform 6 sets of the intermediate version, then bring your feet together so the heels touch and the toes face out. Perform the exercise 8 times in this closed-leg position.

Body Awareness: When you're balancing on your toes, don't let the ankles bow outward, or you'll only weaken them. You can prevent wobbly ankles if you press most of your weight onto the big toes. Squeezing your buttocks and inner thighs together helps to anchor the legs. Be sure your lower back doesn't sway (pull your stomach in). Do you feel the arches, ankles, calves, thighs, and buttocks all working together?

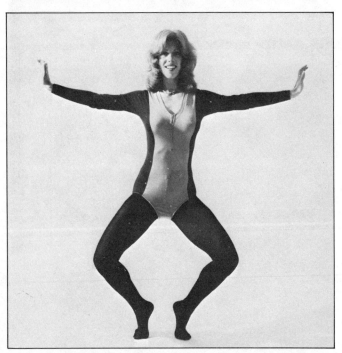

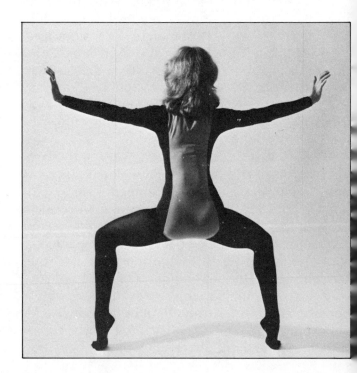

Calf Stretcher

Before-and-after stretch, especially for runners. Since your calf muscles are especially prone to cramping and knotting from jogging, you'll want to develop the habit of stretching them out right before and after your run. Here's one simple way to loosen tight calf muscles. Take your time while you stretch; don't rush your counts.

Position: Face a wall or tree in a lunge position with one foot forward, knee bent—the back foot aligned directly behind it a few paces apart with the knee straight and heel lifted. Elongate your back and extend your arms out to touch the wall.

Beginners: Bounce the back heel up and down to the floor 8 times. If you don't feel the calf muscles stretch each time the back heel touches the floor, then put your legs farther apart. Jump-change legs and repeat the heel bounces with the other leg. Jump-change legs after 8, 4, and 2 bounces per leg without pausing. Relax, then repeat the set.

Intermediates and Advanced: Assume a wider lunge position. Keep both heels flat on the floor. In 4 slow counts, bend just the forward knee as low as possible without lifting your heels. Hold for 4, then straighten on 4. Repeat, then change legs. You may repeat the set as many times as desired on each side until the calf muscles feel loosened.

Body Awareness: For maximum stretch bene-fit, keep the back knee straight and the front knee bent directly over the toes. My beginning students sometimes hunch the shoulders up. Keep them down as you draw the stomach in. This is an expecially good exercise to precede and follow *any* sport or activity that causes the calf muscles to tighten or cramp.

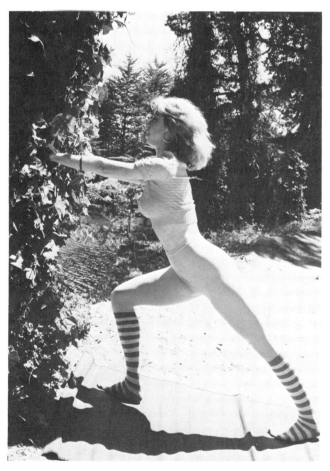

Calf Shaper

Few of us get shapely lower legs from heredity. Slim ankles and contoured calves come from consistent exercise that keep those muscles strong. Here's a simple exercise that you can do at home to improve the muscle tone in your legs and keep them shapely.

Position: Place one foot a pace in front of the other and bend your knees slightly. Let your upper body droop forward with your arms dangling down. Draw your stomach muscles in.

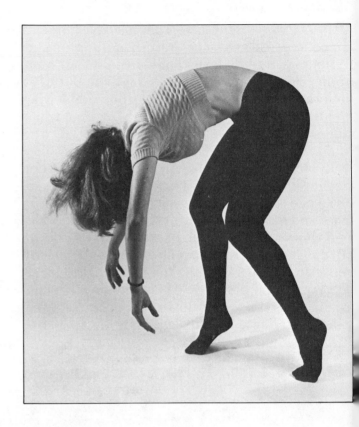

Beginners: In the above position, lift your heels high off the floor and hold them up for 8 slow counts (see photo), then return them to the floor. Repeat 8–10 times, then change the foot position and repeat the set.

Intermediates: Lift your heels while you are dangling forward. Keeping your heels high off the floor, slowly curl up until your back is straight and you are balancing on your toes (take 8 counts to straighten up). Then lower your heels to the floor, drop forward, and repeat. Continue for 5 counts, then change the foot position and repeat for 5 more.

Advanced: Follow the intermediate version until you've curled straight up and you're balancing on your toes. Now, don't let your heels touch the floor. Keep them lifted and slowly lower your upper torso, until you are dangling over as in the starting position. Continue the exercise, without pausing, 3 times. Relax, change feet, and repeat thrice more.

Body Awareness: For most of my students, the difficult part of this exercise is keeping balance. At first you can touch a support, but eventually you should try to balance on your own. If you remember to pull your stomach in and to keep all toes glued to the floor, your balance will also improve.

Foot Rotations

To stretch your feet as you slim the ankles.

Position: Touch the right hand to a wall or support and stand with good posture—flatten your stomach, lengthen your back, and contract your buttocks together, then tuck them under. Think tall. Now stretch the left arm sideways and lift the left foot a few inches off the floor.

Start: Keeping both knees straight, rotate the left foot from the ankle as you describe 8 *slow* circles clockwise. As the foot rotates around, make the toes point down hard and flex up hard so you are really using those foot muscles! Now turn around (left hand on the wall) and continue rotating with the right foot. Repeat both sides once or twice more.

With the left leg out to the side, circle the foot clockwise for 4 counts, then counterclockwise for

4. Without pausing, swing the leg in front of you and continue 4 rotations in one direction, then 4 in the reverse direction. Turn around and repeat with the right foot. Try the sequence a second time without using a support.

Swing the leg from the forward position to directly behind you and continue circling the foot 8 times, reversing direction after every second time. Now turn around and repeat on the other side. Try a second sequence without using the support.

Body Awareness: You're cheating if a knee bends or if you forget any of the 3 posture position checks. For maximum benefit, rotate the foot very slowly. You should be feeling the arch, heel, cord, ankle, and toe muscles all stretching!

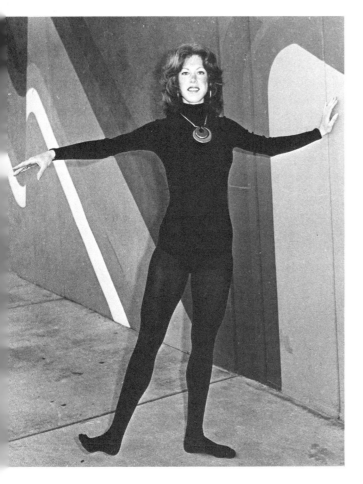
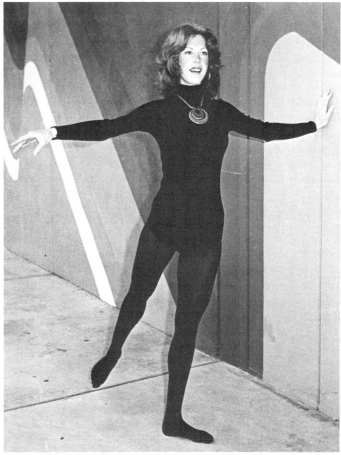

Balancer

Practice your balance and control while you tone the buttocks and thighs and strengthen the feet and ankles.

Position: Stand with heels together and toes opened to the sides: stomach in, back lengthened, buttocks drawn together and tucked under, chest lifted, and shoulder tips pressed down. This is called "dynamic standing."

Beginners: Place one hand on a support or wall. Squeeze the buttocks tightly together so your knees rotate over the toes. As you squeeze, slowly lift your heels off the floor in 4 counts until you are balancing high on the balls of your feet. Hold the balance 4 counts, then gradually lower the heels to the floor in 4 counts. Keep your buttocks contracted throughout the exercise. Repeat 4–6 times before relaxing. Now repeat the exercise 3 times without using a support.

Intermediates: Open your arms to the sides. Perform the beginner exercise twice without a support. For the third repeat, grasp a support and raise both heels high. Now lift the left foot off the floor a few inches with toes pointed. Hold-balance on the right toes 4 counts. Release your support and balance for 4 more counts. Return the left toes to the floor and lower both heels. Repeat the set. Change sides for 2 sets.

Advanced: Perform the beginner exercise twice without holding a support. Open your arms. While the right foot is flat on the floor, raise the left foot to the side a few inches in the air. Point the left toes. Now raise the right heel high and balance for 4 counts. Remain balanced as you bring the left foot to the front for 4 counts, then around to the back for 4 more counts. Now return the left toes to the floor and lower both heels. Relax and repeat the set. Change sides and repeat the set twice.

Body Awareness: If you're losing balance, check your posture position. Remember to keep your buttocks contracted, and to place your weight more toward the big toes. Do you feel the thighs and buttocks toning as the feet and ankles are building strength?

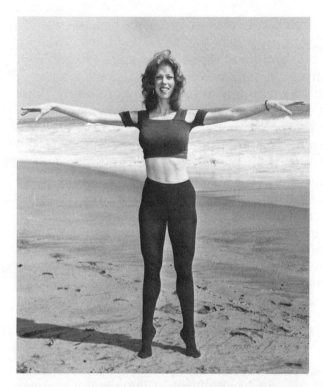

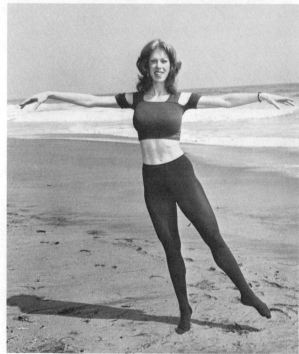

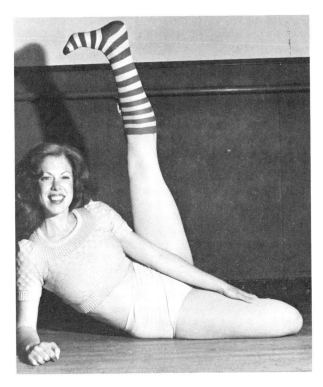

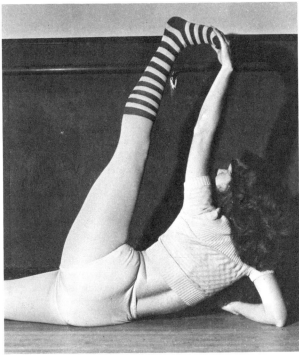

Split-up

Does your job have you standing in one place all day? Do your legs feel stiff after you ski, jog, or play tennis? Do you get a charley horse in your calves after walking up stairs or hilly streets? Most of us are involved in such activities, which keep the calf muscles strong but very tight.

Here's one exercise that not only stretches knotted calves but strengthens and stretches the thigh muscles as well.

Position: Lie on one side and prop yourself up onto your forearm. Bend the leg on the floor at the knee, and straighten the other leg into the air with your foot flexed so that it is parallel to the ceiling. Don't expect to straighten your leg completely!

Beginners: Keeping your knee as straight as possible, gently pulsate your leg toward you 15–20 times. If you're doing this correctly, you'll feel your calf and inner-thigh muscles stretching while your front thigh muscles are building strength. Bend the leg down to relax it, then straighten it up again and repeat the set. Change sides and repeat the exercise twice.

Intermediates: Perform one set of the beginner exercise. Now grasp your leg at the calf and draw it closer to your body. When you've reached your stretch limit, hold the position for 8 counts. Now gently pulsate the leg toward you for 8. Relax the leg, then repeat the entire set. Roll over onto your other side and perform the exercise for 2 sets.

Advanced: Follow the intermediate version, except: you should be grasping your toes while you draw your leg in closer toward your upper torso.

Body Awareness: If you're not feeling a good calf-stretch, then you may not be pushing hard enough through your heel. For extra stretch along the inner thighs, keep your knee very straight. Are you feeling the front thighs getting stronger?

Flexor

Those poor, tired dogs lying down there at the bottom of the heap! What abuse they take—encased in oddly shaped shoes all day, pounded for miles upon hard pavement, and providing the locomotion to allow the superstructure to survive.

Here's an easy foot-stretch that you can do any time during the day to help keep the feet pain-free.

Kick off your shoes and set on the floor or prop your feet up on a stool. Straighten one knee by pointing the toes down very hard.

1. Point the toes of one foot to form a high arch at the instep. Imagine that you're depressing a pedal with your toes, and hold the extreme point position for 5 counts.

2. Now flex just your toes up and back toward you. Feel as though you are pressing the pedal with the bony ridge on the bottom of your foot, and hold for 5.

3. Now flex the foot all the way, so the toes are aimed back toward you and you are pushing hard through your heel. If you push through the heel very hard, and flex the foot way back, your heel will automatically lift off the floor a bit. Hold the extreme flexion for 5 counts. Now try 2 again (half-flexes), then part 1 (point). Continue the three positions several times with the same foot. When it begins to feel looser (after about 5 times), try the exercise (5 times) with the other foot.

Body Awareness: Try to keep the knee of the working foot very straight. If your feet aren't accustomed to being stretched, they may cramp when you point them down. For relief, flex them up immediately as in part 3. Foot cramps are a sign of disuse. Try this exercise daily, any time you can, and you'll soon free your feet from stiffness.

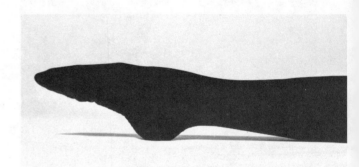

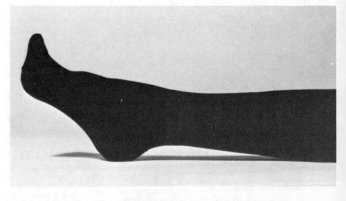

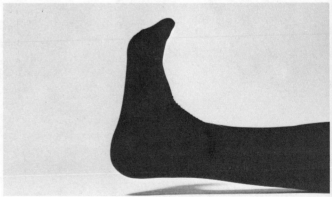

Pebble Pick-up

When you're at the beach in a barefoot condition, try this simple pick-up exercise that helps strengthen your toes and arches for a strong support.

Beginners: Sit surrounded by pebbles (marbles or other small round objects can substitute). Pick up 1 pebble with the toes of your left foot, keeping the heel on the ground. Now twist the toes toward your right foot as far as the foot can pivot, and drop the pebble. Pick it up with the right foot and twist the right foot out, then drop the pebble. Continue with 4 pebbles in this assembly-line fashion, using 4 slow, rhythmic counts to complete the set. Now reverse direction so the right toes begin the pick-up, then twist-drop the foot to the left, etc. Repeat the sequence (4 pebbles in each direction) 2–3 more times.

Intermediate and Advanced: Perform the beginner exercise at a faster rate by increasing the tempo of the sequence, and while standing. After you develop a faster rhythm, try the entire exercise with your eyes closed!

Body Awareness: You cheat if your heels leave the ground. Are you feeling the foot muscles stretching and strengthening? If you feel toe or arch cramps, stop and knead the foot or slap it lightly on the ground until cramps disappear. As your feet are exercised more often, the cramps will diminish. At home, try the entire exercise using marbles.

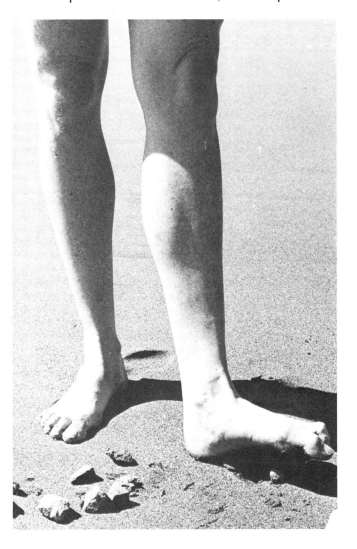
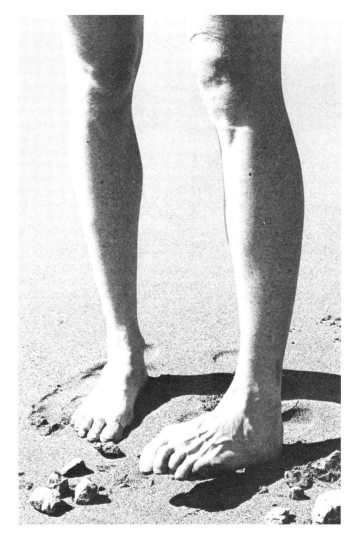

Crisscross Sit-Stand

A lift for sagging arches.

Position: Sit on a chair with the right foot crossed over the left and both arches lifted, so that only the outer borders of your feet are on the floor. Elongate your spine and draw your stomach in. Hands are on your lap.

Beginners: Stand up with your weight on the outer borders of your crossed feet. Try not to lean forward or to use your hands to help you up. Remain standing with the knees straight for 4 counts. Now be seated again, keeping your back straight and your arches lifted. You're cheating if you lean forward when you sit. Repeat, then cross the left foot over the right. Continue the exercise 6–8 times, changing crossed feet after every other set.

Intermediates: Sit on the floor with your legs crossed. Bring your feet in close to you with just the outer borders of the feet on the floor. Now lean forward from your hips and press your hands on the floor to help you stand up. Stand for 4 counts with your knees straight and your weight on the outsides of the feet. Sit down again without moving your feet. Repeat 4–6 times, recrossing your feet after each time you sit.

Advanced: Follow the intermediate version without pressing your hands on the floor to help you up. Instead, clasp your hands behind your back while you stand and sit. Repeat 4–6 times, keeping your weight on the outsides of your feet. Alternate foot-crosses.

Body Awareness: Practice raising to a standing position smoothly and gracefully (and sitting the same graceful way!). In the advanced version, you can lean forward when you raise or sit. You're cheating if the outer borders (from the heel to the little toe) lose contact with the floor.

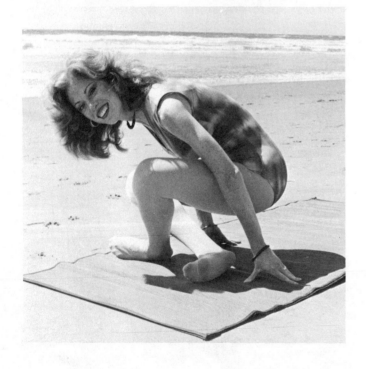
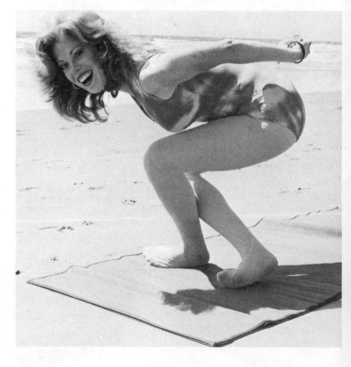

Pre/post-Sports Stretch

A pre-sports stretch helps to keep the muscles flexible, but a post-sports stretch will help to loosen and relax constricted muscles after heavy exercise. Since the calves receive a major workout, you'll want to stretch them before *and* after sports to prevent any painful aftereffects.

Position: Sit on the floor facing a wall, a few inches from it. Both knees are bent. One foot is flat on the floor, and the other foot is pressed flat against the wall. Try to straighten your back.

Beginners and Intermediates: Grasp the ball of the foot that's against the wall with both hands, and pull your toes toward you so that just the heel touches the wall. You may feel a slight stretch along the calf. Still grasping your forefoot, slowly slide your heel higher up along the wall. Your knee will begin to straighten, and you'll begin to feel a stretch along the back of the knee and calf. Slide the heel up the wall as far as your stretch ability allows, then hold this maximum position for 12–16 counts. Return to starting position and repeat. Try the exercise at least 3 times before changing legs. Don't be concerned if your knee won't straighten completely. The point of the exercise is to provide maximum stretch to the calf.

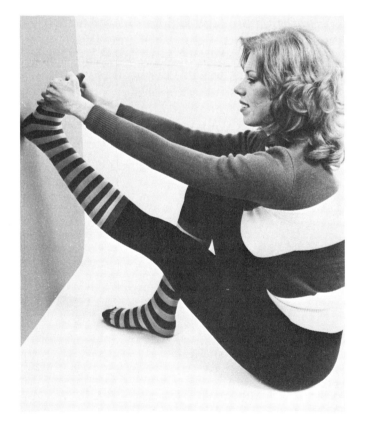

Advanced: You should be able to straighten your knee completely as the heel slides up the wall. Now lift your straightened leg and draw it toward you while you're still grasping the forefoot. Hold it in the air for 16 counts. The closer you draw the leg toward you, the greater stretch you should feel along the calf. Repeat the exercise 2 or more times before changing legs.

Body Awareness: You'll be tempted to round your back as soon as you enter your own calf-stretch zone. Try to keep your back straight and you'll also be lengthening the upper and lower back muscles.

Secret Lower-Leg Exercises
(in public and private places)

• Whenever you're standing at a counter (doing dishes, cooking, brushing teeth) raise up and down on your toes to strengthen the calves, then rock back on your heels to stretch them.

• To strengthen the calves and toes, and to slenderize the ankles, practice walking forward and backward on tiptoe. Even when you can reach for an object without standing on tiptoe, rise up anyway.

• When you're waiting in a line, practice standing with your weight evenly distributed between the heels and balls of the feet (arches lifted).

• If you have "swayback" legs (hyperextended knees that lock backward), practice standing with your weight more toward the front and with your knees relaxed and slightly bent. Any time you're standing (in the shower, brushing your hair, in line, etc.) you can practice the habit of not letting your weight fall onto your heels.

• When you're sauntering down the street, see if you can keep your kneecaps looking straight ahead and aligned over the toes. By controlling the position of the knees you are controlling the position of the ankles too.

• When walking upstairs, don't collapse dependently on the handrail. Instead, use your foot muscles to boost you up by rolling high onto the ball of each foot before taking the next step.

• Practice picking up objects from the floor with your toes by gripping them into little fists.

• Daytime or evening, kick off your shoes and free your toes to stretch. Point them down and flex them up, then rotate them around from the ankles.

• Walking barefoot around the house with your arches lifted will also help keep the calf muscles and heel cord stretched. Practice walking through the house on the outer edges of your feet from time to time.

• Brisk walking (especially barefoot in sand), jogging, jumping, climbing, hiking, running are all great foot and lower-leg exercises. Walk heel to toe, and concentrate on keeping the feet straight, not turned out Charlie Chaplin style or turned in, pigeon-toed.

CHAPTER SEVEN:

SEXY EXERCISES
(For Couples Only)

Are you seeking alternative ways to animate your exercise hour? Try arousing your appetite and enthusiasm for fitness by exercising in accord with another. Substitute a solitary session with some sexy exercises and notice how two toning together tends to turn you on! You'll feel your physical pleasure peak when you perspire with a partner.

I designed sexy exercises for those seeking an additional incentive to their sessions. If you have a tendency to be apathetic about your body, the presence of a partner might motivate you to move. Whether you turn your workout into a sensual, romantic experience with soft lights and music or an energetic, competitive game, your exercise efforts are often improved when you're being watched and helped. With your partner assisting you to stretch farther than you could on your own, or to help you hold a position longer than you would unattended, your progress can be more impressive.

Each of the exercises in this chapter concentrates on a different part of your body in different positions. If you master them all, both of you will be conditioning your muscles for other shared activities. Familiarize yourself with the various couple exercises first; then I encourage you to create a few meaningful duets of your own that will guide you toward your particular physical goals.

Ultimately, a sexy body is supple, strong, and shapely, applying stamina, spirit, and skill to every physical activity. If you want a sexy body, you'll need to develop a consistent conditioning routine based on a variety of exercises from all of the chapters. If you want to share a sensual experience while developing a sexy body, then find a friend and turn this page.

The Technique

Seesaw

Two for the seesaw is a sexy exercise designed to stretch your inner thighs and back while toning your stomach muscles.

Position: Partners sit as closely together as possible with their legs split apart. Point your toes, but don't expect your toes to touch your partner's, especially if he/she has a wider split or longer legs. Grasp hands (or elbows if possible) and straighten your backs so that you're both sitting up high on your haunches.

Seesaw: Begin by lowering your back to the floor while gently pulling your partner toward you. If your partner isn't flexible enough to permit you to touch your back to the floor, then lower yourself only as far as your partner's stretch limit allows. Hold for 6–8 counts before straightening up, then let your partner pull you. Seesaw back and forth very slowly this way several times, striving to touch your backs to the floor as you pull-hold each other.

Body Awareness: While you're lowering your back down to the floor (and pulling your partner with you) do you feel your stomach muscles working? As you curl your back down to the floor, suck in your stomach and feel it building tone and strength.

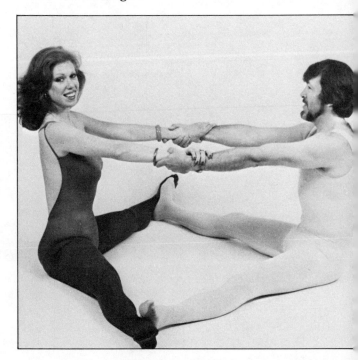

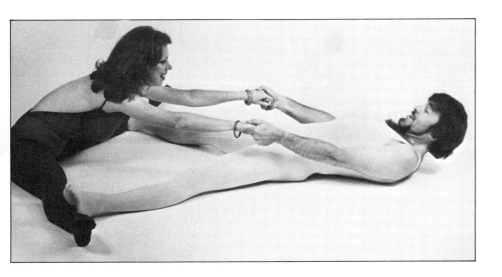

Open-Knee Press

Here's a sexy way to unstiffen your knees and inner thighs and make them flexible.

Position: Lie on your back with knees bent up. Flop them down and open on the floor and bring your soles and heels together, close to your buttocks. Your partner is kneeling at your feet.

Press: Have your partner slowly press your knees down, applying equal and gentle pressure with his/her hands. While your knees are being pressed closer to the floor, try to melt your lower back down by sucking in your stomach. Expect your back to arch a bit despite your effort. As your partner presses your knees down, you'll feel a superstretch along the inner thighs. When you've been pressed to your stretch limit, have your partner hold your knees down there for 5 counts. Then partner raises your knees together to relax them. Repeat the press-hold-relax set 3 times, and notice by the third time how much farther your knees can stretch. Partners change places.

Body Awareness: When pressing on your partner's knees, be sure you do it slowly, with kindness, or you may strain the inner-thigh muscles.

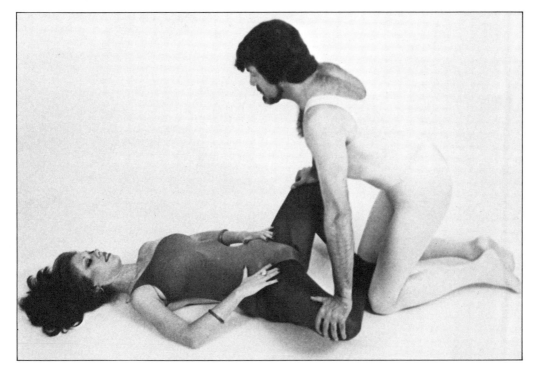

Closed-Knee Press

A gentle back-stretch for both partners simultaneously, although you're in different positions.

Positions: Lie on your back with knees bent up to your chest, and place hands under the neck (or place your arms down at your sides). Your partner stands over you with her/his feet placed next to your hips (knees kept completely straight) and leans over, with the back completely straight and parallel to the floor. Both of you should draw your stomachs in.

While you're relaxing on the floor, standing partner presses your knees closer to your chest until they almost touch your chin. Try to keep hips and lower back on the floor while you hold the pressed position for 10 counts. Relax, then repeat the exercise. Have standing partner gently press and release your knees to your chest for 10 counts.

Meanwhile, if standing partner is keeping the knees straight and back flat, she/he is feeling a superstretch along the back of the thighs and in the lower back.

Partners change places. Repeat this exercise as often as you like.

Body Awareness: Both of you are cheating if you let your stomachs pop out. Be sure your shoulders are relaxed, not hunched up to your ears. Are you both feeling a gentle lower-back stretch?

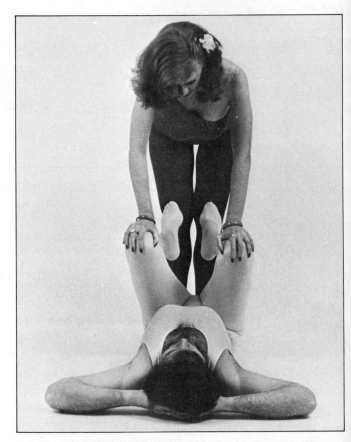

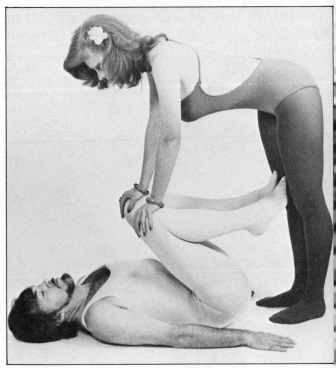

Leg Pulley

A partner can help improve your flexibility better than if you tried to do it yourself. This exercise is a wonderful stretch for the muscles along the inner thighs and for the hamstring muscles in the back of the thighs.

Position: I'm lying on my back with the lower back and shoulders melted into the floor. My working partner stands at my side and raises one of my legs with both his hands.

Very slowly and gently (with kindness) he draws my leg closer toward my upper body. I'm trying to keep *both* of my knees completely straight, with the toes pointed.

If you're working on a beginner or intermediate with somewhat less flexibility, don't expect to be able to push his/her leg too far back. Push it only as far as your partner's limit will allow (a grunt or a few words will let the working partner know when you've reached your stretch limit). Wherever that limit is, hold the leg up and back for 10 counts. Lower the leg to relax it, then immediately bring it up again for a second try. This time strive for a greater stretch.

Change legs and repeat twice, then partners change positions. In the case of a more-advanced partner who has greater flexibility, you can push the leg quite far back before she/he will feel any resistance in the thigh muscles. Count to 10 slowly before releasing the leg.

Body Awareness: You're cheating if you bend the knee of the lifted leg or if you bend the knee that's supposed to be anchored down. Try to keep your back and shoulders flat on the floor. Are you feeling a luxurious stretch along the thigh muscles?

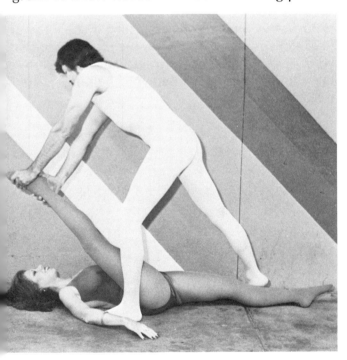

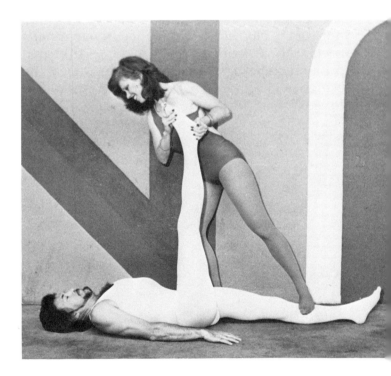

Bosom Butterfly

If you have a tendency toward droopy shoulders, a rounded back, and stiffness in the chest muscles, then let a lover help you out of your slump. This partner exercise trains you to straighten your spine and expand your chest while it helps to relieve upper-back pain and tension in the shoulders.

Position: Sit Indian style on the floor, with back straight and fingers laced behind the neck. The helping partner stands behind the sitting partner and places one knee (bent) in the middle of her/his back for leverage.

Standing Partner: Pull your partner's elbow back as far as possible. Meanwhile, the person seated should be keeping a straight back, with stomach sucked in and head kept as level as possible. Try not to let your head poke forward. When the elbows have been stretched as far back as the seated partner can tolerate, count to 10, then release the elbows (and your knee from partner's back) and let your partner hold the stretched position on his/her own for 10 counts. Repeat the exercise twice more; then partners change places for 3 sets.

Body Awareness: You're cheating if you let your back collapse while you hold the elbows back on your own. Also, try not to let your knees move even the slightest bit when your helping partner releases your elbows.

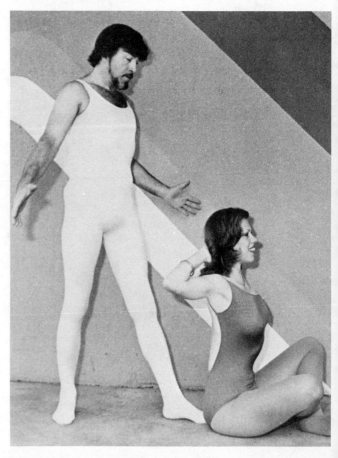

Two-timing Waist Twist

Some people call it "love handles," others refer to it as their "spare tire," and a few sigh "ring around my rosy." When that incisive wedge-shaped midriff turns into a ball of puffed pastry, you can begin to comprehend how sedentary living can literally run circles around you. A combination of diet and exercise can reduce the rim around the middle, but exercise is the essential ingredient to maintain the tone.

This new twist for two stretches out your waist like it's never been stretched before. Fair warning: This exercise looks easy enough, but it's really quite memorable if you do it correctly.

Working Partner: Lie on your back with your hands laced under your neck and your knees bent up to your chest. Have your helping partner kneel above your head and press your elbows down so they are anchored to the floor.

Now *slowly* lower your knees to one side of your body and touch the floor. Take it easy. Be sure legs are glued tightly together as they twist over to one side. Hold the position for 4 slow counts, then lift the knees for 4 and continue to lower them over to the other side on the floor. Hold for 4, then bring them up again. Continue rotating legs from side to side for 4 or more sets while your helping partner is pressing your elbows down. Partners change positions and repeat the entire exercise.

Body Awareness: If you haven't been doing good waist-stretches in a while, at first you won't be able to keep your knees together or at waist height when you twist them from side to side. Lower the knees but keep them together. As ability improves, try twisting with your knees held higher. If you're doing this exercise correctly, you should be feeling a superstretch, starting along the sides of your waist and running all the way up your underarm. You'll need to use your stomach muscles to lift your knees from side to side.

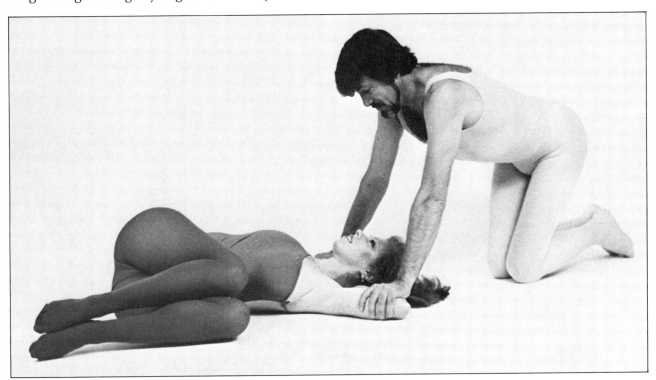

Couple Curl-down

Two together can tone a flabby abdomen effectively.

Position: Partners sit facing each other with legs about shoulder-width apart and bent slightly at the knees. Hook your feet under each other's thighs or knees for leverage, and straighten your spine so you are both sitting as tall as possible. Reach your arms overhead and draw in your stomach.

Start: In 4 slow counts, you both curl your back down toward the floor, stopping at a point where your lower back almost touches the floor. Hold this suspended position for 8 counts, then curl back up on 8. Repeat the exercise without pausing—until one of you gives up!

Body Awareness: You're cheating if you rush the counts, or if you let your stomach protrude during any part of the exercise. When you return to starting position, remember to lengthen the spine completely before descending again.

You should really feel those abdominal muscles building strength! Are you also feeling the thigh and hip muscles strengthening?

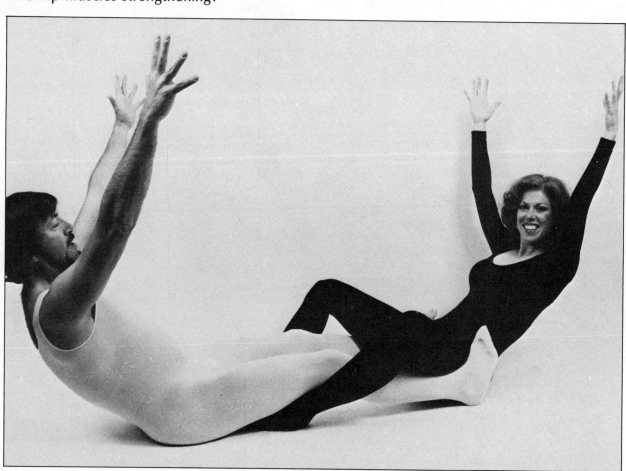

Partner Payoff

CAUTION: *Consult your doctor first if you have low-back pain.*

A partner is helping you tone the buttocks and strengthen the lower back.

Working partner gets down on all fours with elbows straight and head up. Let your helping partner raise one leg up high behind you. When your leg has been lifted to its height limit, helping partner releases your leg and *you* hold it up on your own for 8 slow counts. You're cheating if the leg drops in height after your partner releases it! Lower and change legs.

Repeat the entire sequence a second time, trying to hold each leg high for more than 8 counts, then kick it up for 8 counts. Now switch positions and help your partner with this exercise.

Body Awareness: Be sure that your lifted leg is very straight (no bent knee allowed), and your toes are pointed. Try to keep your chest and hips from twisting sideways when one leg is raised. Do you feel those muscles in the buttocks and lower back building strength?

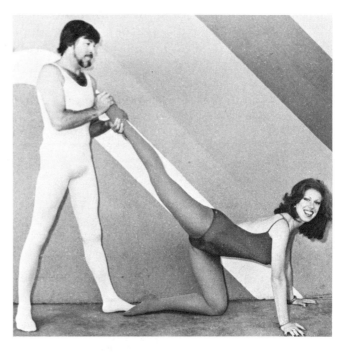

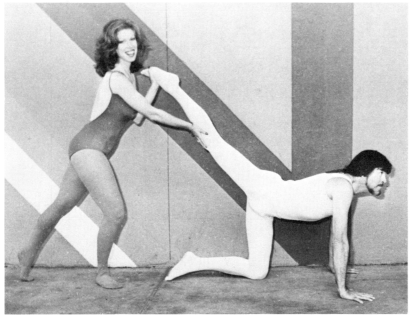

A Pressing Encounter

Here is one example of how to combine two distinct exercises into one harmonious combination. The Plow (Chapter Three) is combined with Isometric Push-ups (Chapter Five) into an intimate encounter.

The partner on top strengthens arms and chest with push-ups while the partner on the floor stretches back and hamstring muscles in the plow position. Partners change places before either is too fatigued.

Try this combination first, then create a few of your own. Good luck!

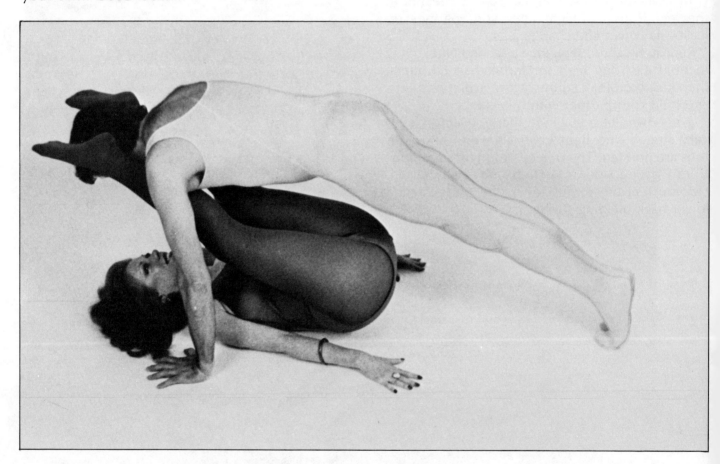

Buddy Back Bend

> CAUTION: *Back bends are not for people with low-back problems.*

Some exercises seem threatening until you try them with a buddy. Then you discover that with a pair of helping hands, your body can manage to bend into positions you thought were impossible. I've discovered many with a fear of doing back bends because of the upside-down position this exercise takes. But a buddy can give you confidence.

Position: Lie on the floor with your palms down next to your ears, knees bent up, and feet on the floor, about shoulder-width apart. Helping partner stands over you and grasps you with both hands at your lower back, gently lifting you in the middle. Meanwhile you are pressing hands and feet evenly into the floor, letting your head drop back, and arching your back up. You may feel a stretch along the stomach area while being held in this backbend position.

From here, have your partner hold you up for 10 counts before letting you down. Try this exercise a second time. On the third try, have helping partner step away while you hold the back-bend position on your own.

When you become better at this, have helping partner hold you up while you deepen your back arch by walking the hands and feet closer together! Now ask your partner to step away while you hold this deeper back bend.

Body Awareness: You should be feeling a wonderful stretch up the abdomen to the neck and shoulders while you sense the arms, back, and legs exerting strength. In addition to being a good upper-body stretch, this exercise also helps to strengthen the arms, chest, and upper back. Now change places with your buddy.

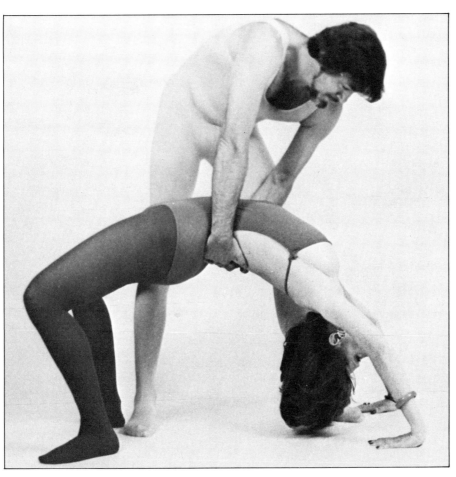

Joint Back-up

CAUTION: *Not for people with back problems.*

With a little help, you can strengthen the lower back and buttocks while stretching the abdominal and chest muscles.

Position: Lie face down with your feet a few inches apart and your fingers laced behind your neck. Helping partner kneels behind you and firmly anchors your feet to the floor.

The Back-up: In one fast count, lift your chest up and arch your back as high as possible off the floor. Hold the back-up position for 8 slow counts—without dropping in height! Meanwhile, partner has a firm anchor on your feet. Return to the floor and relax. Repeat the exercise twice more, each time arching higher off the floor. Change partners, so that you each have a chance to work your backs.

Body Awareness: Squeeze buttocks together when you arch your back up. When holding the position on your own, are you feeling those back muscles building strength?

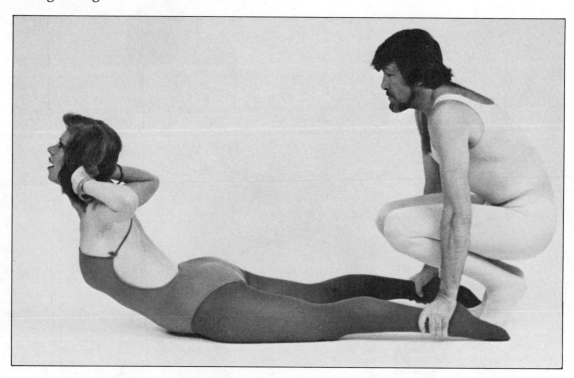

Playing Footsies

Here's one of my favorite foot exercises, which is guaranteed to relax your whole body and bring relief to downtrodden feet. Done with a little TLC, this exercise will feel like a sensual foot massage. Then feel free to add a few touches of your own!

Position: Sit on the floor with legs stretched out long, knees straight and toes pointed. Your partner is kneeling at your feet.

Start: Partner grasps one of your feet with both hands in such a way that the palms are on top and the fingers are wrapped under the instep. Very slowly, partner presses palms on the foot, arching and stretching it down toward the floor. Meanwhile, you must keep your knees completely straight. Indicate to your partner when your foot has been stretched to its maximum. At that point,

partner holds the stretched position for 8 counts. Be sure you don't cry "Help!" until you really feel a stretch. Next, partner will reverse the stretch by flexing your foot up so that the toes are aimed toward you. Partner repeats this exercise two or three more times, then does the same to your other foot.

Now it's your turn to treat your partner to the same stretch on both feet!

Body Awareness: For this foot stretch to be effective, be sure the toes are in line with the knee when your partner presses down on your foot. Don't let the toes turn in or twist out. You're cheating if the knee bends. Smile—this is really a luxurious foot stretch that should also help you to relax.

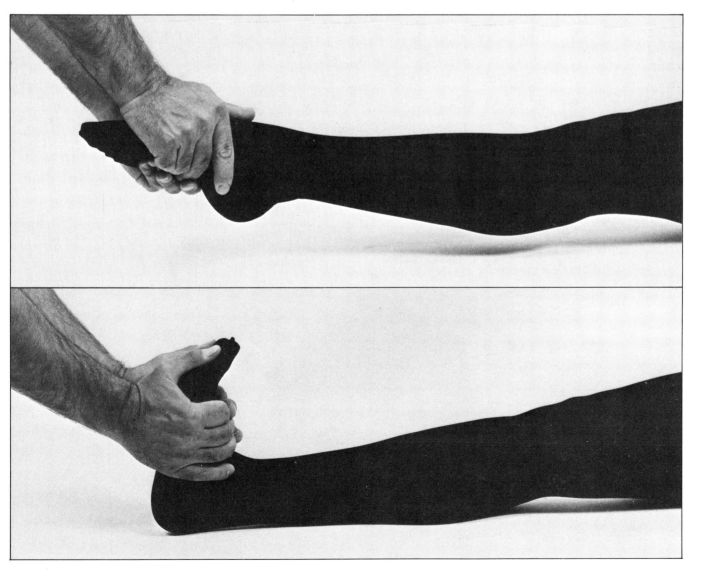

CHAPTER EIGHT:

HOW'S YOUR HEART AND DIET?

Spark Your Heart

No body-conditioning or exercise program can be complete if it's designed to develop the skeletal muscles only. Since the most important muscle-organ in your body is the heart, to neglect it in an exercise program is to neglect your very lifeline! Like all muscles, the heart increases in size, and strength, and efficiency when exercised, or becomes weak when unexercised. Athletes, for example, have the strongest, largest hearts; sedentary adults have the smallest, softest hearts. Coronary attacks are twice as prevalent among the sedentary middle aged than the physically active. Although there are several risk factors contributing to heart attacks—heredity, age, sex, stress, high cholesterol levels, and high blood pressure—through exercise you can directly decrease at least the last two factors.

An efficient, healthy heart is made to work harder through gradual but consistent exercise. By strengthening it you improve its ability to pump blood to the muscles and increase the blood-oxygen supply to the muscles and the brain. The less-efficient, less-exercised heart can't move as much blood with each beat. Thus the brain and muscles receive less nourishment.

By exercising you can develop a collateral circulatory system—a growth of new blood vessels and capillaries in the muscles being used. When you increase the blood flow to your muscles, you get a "high"; you feel energized because nourishment and oxygen are filling the cells. The cells are left partly empty when you're sitting around; the oxygen supply is diminished, and you begin to feel a sedentary fatigue. To keep the vessels open and filled, your heart must be made to work!

Exercises that improve the cardiovascular system are called isotonics, aerobics, or dynamic exercises. They involve continuous, rhythmic, and repetitive movements that are sustained over a period of time lasting *at least* 4 minutes. Heart-conditioning exercises are those that involve large muscle groups; they make you sweat freely and breathe hard. They make your lungs sing. They're the more vigorous exercises that keep more muscles moving for a longer time. Jumping rope, running, jogging, bike-riding, swimming, fast dancing, brisk walking, and most rhythmic movements that are repeated till you are sweaty are all excellent cardiovascular conditioners. In my technique I have you jump rope and do jumping exercises for the feet, which also condition your heart (such as Pinwheels). Exercises that cannot be sustained for at least 3 minutes (i.e., sprinting) won't benefit your heart.

Always check with your doctor before starting cardiovascular exercise. If you have his clearance, begin conditioning the heart as you would your skeletal muscles. Start the activity gradually, in small doses, and perform the exercise or sport consistently (at least three times per week). Aim for a reasonable amount of deep respiration and perspiration, but please stop before you reach exhaustion or breathlessness. To derive maximum benefit for the cardiovascular system, try to sustain your chosen activity for 15–20 minutes. (Equate 1 minute of jumping rope with 3 minutes of jogging.)

The heart and lungs are most involved in activities that call upon vigorous, continuous use of your skeletal muscles. When you increase the use of these muscles, you're exercising the heart even more. Isolated or "spot" conditioning exercises (i.e., stomach strengtheners, leg stretches, etc.), although very important and necessary for toning and flexibility, usually do not provide enough activity to benefit your heart muscle. That's why brisk walking, jumping rope, jogging, sports, or fast dancing are a necessary part of your total conditioning program.

As with all exercise, precede a cardiovascular activity with a warm-up session. When the capillaries and blood vessels in the muscles are at rest, they don't have a full blood supply. By gradually increasing the movements of your muscles, you'll increase the blood flow to their capillaries. For a muscle to function at its optimum level of ability, it must have a full and constant blood supply. In the warm-up period, you're merely arousing (not shocking) your muscles so that they can gather energy from the increased blood flow and be better prepared for more strenuous activity. You're also working your heart by increasing the demand on it to pump more blood to the working muscles at a faster rate.

Follow a long, vigorous workout with a 5-minute (or more) cool-down period. Slowly wind down your activity so the blood can continue circulating, but at a slower rate. Abruptly stopping after 15 minutes or more of an energetic workout can cause dizziness, fainting, or nausea.

Everyone has a maximum point at which the heart can't beat any faster to deliver more oxygen and blood to the muscles. To prolong exercising beyond this maximum is to approach exhaustion. We also have a minimum rate at which the heart must beat to exercise and condition it. One method used to indicate if you are exercising at your maximum aerobic ability is to take your pulse immediately upon stopping the exercise. The most beneficial pulse rates lie between 70 and 85 percent of your maximum ability, which varies for everyone depending on age, heredity, and fitness level. To figure your desirable level of heartbeats per minute, subtract your age from 220, then find 70 percent and 85 percent of that number. For example, at age 30: 30 from 220 equals 190; 70 percent of that is 133; 85 percent is 162. The pulse rate of a 30-year-old should be between 133 and 162 during a 15–30-minute cardiovascular exercise session.

You can check your pulse to see if it lies within the 70–85-percent range by stopping periodically and immediately counting your heartbeats for 6 seconds, then multiplying that number by 10. "Immediately" is the key word here, because after 6 seconds of inactivity your heartbeat begins to drop rapidly and your pulse reading won't be accurate. If your reading lies above or below your desirable range, then you are working your heart over or under its most efficient level. Checking your pulse rate can be conveniently accomplished with a stopwatch when walking briskly, jogging, or jumping rope, but not when involved in sports! Its purpose is to help you develop an awareness of when you're exercising the heart to its greatest benefit. Personally, I find the pulse-taking method an annoyance and an interruption. Try it once, but really, you should be able to sense when you're overexerting or underexerting yourself without taking your pulse.

As the heart becomes better conditioned, the resting pulse rate will lower. You'll then need to increase the intensity or duration of your workout to keep the pulse rate in the 70–85-percent range; that is, you're sweating freely and breathing deeply.

Maintaining your cardiovascular system in good condition requires a commitment of at least three 15–20-minute vigorous exercise sessions per week. If you discontinue the activity for longer than a month's time, expect to begin again from the very beginning!

When exercising your heart muscle, you're also making the lungs more efficient by forcing them to expand and accommodate the body's need for a greater supply of fresh oxygen. The extent of the body's need for oxygen (and need to eliminate carbon dioxide) will determine automatically the rate and depth of your breathing. If you're involved in an energetic activity (i.e., jogging) your breathing will automatically be more rhythmic, deeper, and heavier than if you're doing some gentle stretching exercises. The only rule about breathing is to *let it happen naturally*; never force it or interfere with it. Trust your lungs; they've known how to inhale and expel air from birth, they never needed your mind to direct them. Forced deep breathing, especially when there is no physical activity to warrant it, will only cause dizziness or fainting. You don't need to force yourself to inhale and exhale in a conscious, controlled way while exercising; it only distracts you from the important consideration of the exercise itself—how the muscles are being used. Just remember to keep your lips parted so that you can breathe naturally through your mouth. Entrust the breathing process to your lungs; they are designed to accommodate from birth the oxygen needs of your body!

As heart and lung conditioners, most sports are excellent, because they keep you active for a long period of time. They also help to develop coordination. A few sports, such as golf, bowling, or backyard Ping-Pong, although helpful in developing coordination, won't place enough demand on your cardiovascular system to benefit it.

Sports provide an enjoyable way to exercise, but they have their limitations. They're rarely performed daily, and they don't exercise the body parts equally. In fact, some sports develop asymmetry or postural defects. Tennis and baseball, for example, develop muscles in only one arm—and since the basic waiting position for the ball is stooped, rounded shoulders develop. Jogging improves the heart and lung capacity and strengthens the legs, but it ignores the arms, chest, shoulders, neck, and coordination. Swimming does not make supple, flexible back and hamstring muscles. Hatha yoga postures *do* increase flexibility, but do not strengthen the skeletal muscles, and they ignore the heart muscle. Sports in themselves won't develop your body as well as an overall concentrated conditioning program.

From the preceding pages, you may realize that a strong, fluid, coordinated, radiant body can be designed and hewn through a persistent, intelligent, and effective exercise program. By incorporating cardiovascular activity, we can know the feeling of living in an alive body!

Diet Tips

Every so often all of us need to take a body inventory and evaluate our diet. Has your wedged waist reshaped itself into a perfect rectangle? Are you starting to decorate what you can no longer hide? Have you tried dieting for three weeks and only lost 21 days? Are you sick of counting calories, carbohydrates, glasses of water, or grams?

According to the latest U.S. Public Health Service estimates, at least one-quarter to one-half of the adult population of this country are more than 20 percent overweight due to overeating and under-exercising. At the moment there are as many diets and diet aids as there are ice-cream flavors, and each diet has its own list of testimonials, books, and special-ingredient products. Whether you allow yourself to be starved, shocked, modified, amphetamined, or hypnotized into losing weight, beware, since the costs and recidivism rates of diet fads are high. Only the strong-willed survive. The fact remains that over 10 billion dollars was spent last year by overweight Americans who wanted to wear a bikini by summer. The deliberate self-deprivation that 70 million Americans suffer due to prior caloric overindulgence has become a national obsession.

Let's be sensible for a moment and review a few basic facts about diet and exercise and their effects on the body. Quite simply, if you *consume* more food than you use up in a day, an excess of fat will be stored in your body. If you *use* more food (exercise) than you consume, then you will lose some of the stored fat. So the only way to lose weight is to consume less, exercise more, or a combination of both.

If you lose weight without exercising, you'll be a thin person with loose sections of hanging flab on your body . . . like a tapering candle with dripping wax. The looseness won't be due to stored fat, but to slack muscles that have lost their tone. Only exercise can tone those sections. If you decide to exercise without watching your diet, you can develop into a toned bulldozer. Weight loss through exercise is a very slow process: It takes 10 minutes to jog off four ounces of champagne; 18 minutes to swim off one small slice of holiday fruitcake.

Exercise is really an *aid* to weight reduction, not a method of losing weight *per se*. Dieting is for those who are thick and tired of it. You reduce your weight by dieting; you firm your form by exercising your softwear.

One sophisticated method of determining how thick you are (the amount of body fat you have) is by a skin-fold test. Calipers measure the thickness of folds of skin at selected spots on your body, and the percentage of body fat is then calculated. If you have more than 30 percent body fat, you're considered to be obese. Personally, my favorite easy method is the "pinch test." Half of your body fat is right under the skin, so if you can pinch more than one inch of skin and fat in any area, then that area needs exercise, and maybe a diet as well.

Women inherit more stored fat than men: A woman's body is about 25 percent fat; a man's is about 12 percent fat. The length and thickness of our bones are also inherited, resulting in basic differences in body build (somatype). By exercising we can enlarge the size of the muscles, but women don't show the bulk. Men show bulging muscles because of their thinner layer of stored fat. Of course, no amount of exercise will change the actual length and thickness of the bones. You can be a big-boned thin person or a small-boned obese person. Your basic somatype isn't nearly as important as what you've done with it in terms of diet and exercise.

Quite honestly, I always feel a bit uncomfortable giving general advice regarding what a person should or should not eat. There are too many individual variables—taste preferences, psychological dependence on food, allergies, etc.—for me to make one general diet recommendation for all readers. There are, however, some diet *tips* I'd like to share with you. Whenever you get food cravings, munch all you want on everything you don't like. Think slow, small, fresh, and balanced. In other words, take a *long* time eating *small* portions of fresh (not canned) foods, and eat a variety from every group except refined sugar and saturated fats. Learn to think of candy, sugary desserts, and deep-fried foods as poison to your precious body. True, you may choose to poison yourself occasionally, but treat healthy foods with the same respect you give to a chocolate mousse. Start thinking of fresh, juicy fruit as a delicious, delectable dessert treat.

By cutting down on food, you don't necessarily cut down on all your friends and relatives who make it. You just don't eat the same *quantities* as before, because you're now imagining yourself to be a thinner person who doesn't need so much anymore.

Convince yourself that you're stuffed when you're feeling satisfied, not full. And you don't need to handle pressure or settle arguments in the kitchen with the refrigerator door wide open, either. If you can't stand the heat (frustration), get *out* of the kitchen. It's very tempting to use food to fill psychological needs: as a comfort when we're upset, as a great escape, as a rich and immediate reward, as a sensual pleasure, as a filler of loneliness, or as a means of procrastinating a distasteful task. Dealing with personal problems without food requires behavior modification and tremendous will power.

It takes lots of will power to give up trying to diet, too! By resolving to reshape a rectangular waist into a whittled wedge, you need not starve, deprive, or punish yourself. Remember only one simple rule: Eat less and move more, for now and forever after!

CHAPTER NINE:

THE LUSTGARTEN TECHNIQUE

The Lustgarten Technique of Dynamic Body Conditioning is an original, well-researched, well-tested system of exercises. I have created and developed it during six years of teaching and researching and ten years of active experience with dance and athletics. The technique conditions all muscles safely, effectively, comprehensively, and rhythmically (to music) without the use of equipment or apparatus.

The Technique uses any of four different exercise formats that you can do at home. In the following pages I've summarized Format 2. Each format lasts about 45–60 minutes and uses about 30 exercises from the previous chapters, arranged into a logical sequence to help you avoid injury. Each format has its own music tape. Music is a vital part of my Technique because it sets an inspiring mood and rhythm. I've carefully selected disco, jazz, and blues that provide just the right rhythm and feeling for each exercise in sequence (Formal 2 also has an accompanying instruction and music tape).

If you carefully follow any of the four formats, your fabulous body will be receiving maximum conditioning benefits: 53 strengtheners, 54 stretches, 2 different cardiovascular conditioners, 7 coordination challenges, 5 different balances, and 45–60 minutes of posture work! Additionally, you'll be rescuing your body-mind from sedentary fatigue and tension; and you'll be preconditioning your muscles with the basic vocabulary for sports, sex, and fashion.

Once your doctor gives you clearance, I recommend performing the Technique three to four times per week, every other day at first. You should see and feel improvement after only four weeks. Don't try the advanced exercises until the intermediate version is too comfortable. For tips on getting started, review the introduction.

To me, a dynamic body is one that combines science with art: balance, coordination, and grace combined with strength and stamina. Mere strength or flexibility is not enough to make your body a dynamic one. Posture plays an important part in keeping the body balanced and graceful. A well-placed and centered body has no sense of stress or strain in the muscles. The total feel is one of weightlessness and of free-and-easy movement.

Think of your body as made up of separate building blocks, each one balanced over the other. If your alignment is correct, the centers of gravity of these units will be lined up with the center of your body, and the parts will be held together by strong muscles. But if a "block" slips off-center due to habit or a weakened muscle, then other blocks will shift to compensate. This crooked alignment may still hold together, but very precariously. Gravity now exerts its pull along the edges of the shifted parts (i.e., round shoulders, saggy stomach) and the weakened muscles begin to strain in their attempt to prevent the drooped parts from tumbling. This off-center placement is what eventually causes your muscles to ache.

In our bodies, the center of gravity lies just below the navel. When the blocks are well-aligned under and over the navel, the body is stabilized. We balance easier if the center is supported by muscular strength in the stomach and lower back. We lose balance when we're misaligned or when the muscles are too weak to hold the center over the base of support.

Since balance is so important, not only in my Technique but in any physical endeavor, why not try these posture-correction hints right now, while you're reading. Stand in front of a mirror and think regal (*not* military). Begin by drawing your stomach (abdominal muscles) in and up. Imagine that your belly button is an elevator button. If you press the button in and ride the elevator up one flight, you'll be making the correct adjustment! Your chest will also elevate slightly so that it just "floats" atop your stomach. Continuing up, feel your shoulders relax down with the blades drawn back slightly, but not pinched so far back that your chest marches forward. Level out your shoulders if they don't seem even, and let your arms hang loosely. Now you'll want to look straight out from a head that's perched on a lengthened neck, nose pointed into the future. Congratulations. At this point you've lengthened your spine, grown an inch in height, and lost an inch in girth!

Now for your lower half. Squeeze your buttock and upper-thigh muscles together, then tuck hips under slightly (imagine you're tucking your tail under you). By squeezing and tucking, you're helping to straighten out the lower-back curve, and are supporting the lower-back muscles. Drawing your stomach in helps to accomplish the same. Your knees should have the same relaxed bend as do the elbows; don't lock them back tightly. Finally, feel your lifted and balanced body weighted evenly on both feet. The weight should pass down the center of your lifted arches, with pressure points felt equally on the balls and heels. In your elongated and balanced state, try to look dynamically relaxed. Smile.

Do you feel some uncomfortable strains? Over the years, misalignments and imbalances can become comfortable habits, making any correction feel awkward and jarring. The farther out of alignment your muscle parts have slipped, the more uncomfortable these corrections will seem.

Most postural faults come from bad habits and unconditioned muscles. As muscles are allowed to lose their tone, they don't hold our body erect. If the downward pull of gravity becomes stronger than our efforts to remain straight, then gravity's pull will round our shoulders down, sink the chest in, droop the head forward, and tug on the abdominal muscles so that all the abdomen's contents spill against a sagging, protruding abdominal wall. What a deteriorating mess! No wonder we experience stress, strain, tension, fatigue, backaches, headaches, even constipation, indigestion, and foot cramps!

There's another reason why I incorporate alignment into my Technique. Posture is the most expressive and dynamic part of our appearance. Whatever self-image we hold—confident or depressed, alert or bored, winner or loser—it is immediately reflected in a proud or lubberly carriage. What's the point of exercising to stretch and strengthen the muscles if we're oafish in our daily movements? Without attention to alignment, there can be no harmony within a body. By concentrating on posture, we can produce the graceful, elegant carriage that we were always meant to have.

Once you try my conditioning Technique, you'll notice that coordination is another element I've incorporated. Coordination is measured by movements that are performed with skill and control. Many muscle groups synchronize at just the precise moment. Your muscles receive their signals from the brain via nerve impulses, which activate certain groups to contract and stabilize while others are relaxing. With conscious practice, your muscles can be trained to synchronize (contract-relax) efficiently. The more highly developed the muscles, the more refined their movements as they coordinate and the more efficient and precise their performance becomes. When your movements become economical, you look graceful and harmonious.

Don't expect weak muscles to have the capability of stabilizing or coordinating skillfully enough to deliver an accomplished performance. When weak muscles hold the body parts in disarray, an activity becomes difficult and awkward to perform, and movements are jerky and gross instead of smooth and refined. More energy is expended than is necessary to accomplish the movement, causing the muscles to poop out early.

Perfect neuromuscular control takes conscious practice and training to learn where to place the muscles during separate, simple movements. Eventually we discover that posture, balance, and coordination are interdependent, orchestrating to create a harmonious whole. We begin to feel an aesthetic pleasure in moving skillfully. The final result should appear to be a symphony of seemingly effortless perfection in motion.

In developing the exercise formats and music tapes, I hoped to present this comprehensive fitness technique in a joyful, entertaining, and spirited way. We all should feel exhilarated while watching our bodies become beautiful. Have fun with it! Good luck!

The Lustgarten Technique, Format 2

TIME (min:/sec)	EXERCISES	PAGE
5:00	1. Jumping Rope (to music)	
4:30	2. Sidewinder or Windmill Lunge	
	3. Warm-up or Half Bounces	
	4. Warm-up or Full Bounces	
4:30	5. Roof-Plié Reach	
	6. Rib-Cage Isolation (Standing)	
	7. Pinwheels	
5:30	8. Diamond Knee Bends	
	9. Parallel Knee Bends	
	10. Heel-ups	
	11. Balancer	
7:00	12. Sidekicks (with balance)	
	13. Kickbacks (with balance)	
	14. Rover's Revenge	
	15. Easy Thigh-Stretcher	
	16. Sprinter	
	17. Sidesprint	
6:30	18. Partner Seesaw	
	19. Pretzel Twist	
	20. Pretzel Reach	
	21. Long Stretch Forward	
5:00	22. Scissors (with bent knees)	
	23. Small Bridge (with bounce)	
	24. Backbend Bridge	
	25. Lying Leg Pulls	
	26. Plow (optional)	
3:00	27. Snail	
	28. Kneeling Push-downs	
4:00	29. Shoulder Rolls and Oppositions	
	30. Neck Rolls	
	31. Partner Foot Stretch	

Total: 45 minutes

ABOUT THE AUTHOR

Karen Lustgarten is a national best-selling author and a newspaper columnist. Her exercise column, "The Dynamic Body," has appeared weekly in the *San Francisco Chronicle* since 1975, and was syndicated for a year. The "Secret Exercises" segments that she created, produced, and performed for television earned her a Northern California Emmy Award nomination. She has also written a television program devoted to health and fitness. Classes in her technique were conducted in San Francisco. Karen now resides in Los Angeles, where she makes television appearances and does fitness and dance consulting.

ABOUT THE LUSTGARTEN TAPES

Since the Lustgarten Technique uses music, each of the four exercise formats is accompanied by a different music cassette tape. Formats 1 and 2 last 45 minutes; Formats 3 and 4 last 60 minutes.

If you wish to purchase a tape, please indicate the numbered format you desire: *music with written instructions* are available for Formats 1–4. Format 2 also has a spoken instruction tape available for purchase.

Send $10 per tape. Make check or money order payable to:

Lustgarten
P.O. Box 3757
Los Angeles, California 90028

Include your name, address, and phone number with your order.